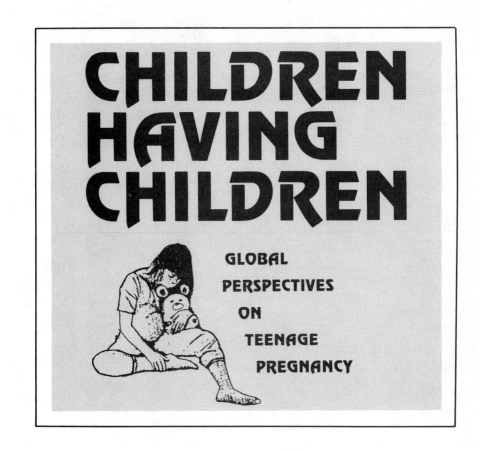

CHILDREN HAVING CHILDREN

GLOBAL PERSPECTIVES ON TEENAGE PREGNANCY

Gary E. McCuen

IDEAS IN CONFLICT SERIES

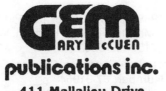

GEM

GARY McCUEN

publications inc.

411 Mallalieu Drive
Hudson, Wisconsin 54016

Illustrations & Photo Credits
Craig MacIntosh 65, Star Tribune 93, Eleanor Mill 119, 124, David Seavey 101, 113, 129.

© 1988 by Gary E. McCuen Publications, Inc.
411 Mallalieu Drive ● Hudson, Wisconsin 54016
(715) 386-5662

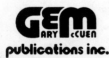

Library of Congress Catalog Card
Number: 87-91954
International Standard Book Number 0-86596-064-X
Printed in the United States of America

CONTENTS

Ideas in Conflict   6

CHAPTER 1   GLOBAL PERSPECTIVES ON ADOLESCENT PREGNANCY

1 U.S. TEEN PREGNANCY RATES ARE FALLING   9
   Eleanor J. Bader
2 THE RATES ARE RISING   15
   General Accounting Office
3 ADOLESCENT FERTILITY: 23
   WORLDWIDE CONCERNS
   Judith Senderowitz and John M. Paxman
4 ADOLESCENT FERTILITY IN NIGERIA   33
   The Pathfinder Fund
5 TEENAGE PREGNANCY IN SCOTLAND   40
   Family Planning Perspectives
6 PREGNANCY RATES IN THE CARIBBEAN   44
   Tirbani B. Jagdeo
7 TEENAGE SEXUALITY AND PREGNANCY   48
   IN AUSTRALIA
   Stefania Siedlecky
8 EARLY PREGNANCY IN BRAZIL AND   53
   GUATEMALA
   Marilyn Edmunds and John M. Paxman

CHAPTER 2   PREVENTING TEENAGE PREGNANCY

9 SEX EDUCATION HAS FAILED   60
   William J. Bennett
10 SEX EDUCATION HAS NOT FAILED   68
   Karen Sue Smith
11 CONTRACEPTIVES AND THE RISE IN   76
   PREGNANCIES: POINTS AND
   COUNTERPOINTS
   Howard Hurwitz vs. The Nation

12 SCHOOL BASED CLINICS WILL NOT WORK   81
    Phyllis Schlafly
13 SCHOOL CLINICS CAN REDUCE   89
    PREGNANCY RATES
    Laurie S. Zabin, Marilyn B. Hirsch, Edward A.
    Smith, Rosalie Streett, and Janet B. Hardy
14 REMOVING ADVERTISING RESTRICTIONS   96
    ON CONTRACEPTIVES
    The Population Institute
15 CONTRACEPTIVE COMMERCIALS ARE   103
    INAPPROPRIATE
    Alfred R. Schneider
16 DECEIVING OURSELVES ABOUT SAFE SEX   108
    Anthony B. Robinson

CHAPTER 3   PREGNANCY AMONG BLACK TEENAGERS

17 THE VANISHING MALE CHARACTER   115
    Michael Novak
18 BLAMING THE VICTIM   120
    Chris Booker
19 AN AGENDA FOR SOCIAL REFORM   125
    Marian Wright Edelman
20 TOWARD A SOCIALIST FUTURE   135
    Angela Davis and Fania Davis

CHAPTER 4   TEENAGE PREGNANCY: IDEAS IN CONFLICT

21 SOCIETY PROMOTES TEENAGE PREGNANCY   145
    Therman E. Evans
22 THE INDIVIDUAL IS RESPONSIBLE   151
    Joseph W. Tkach
23 CHASTITY AND SELF-DISCIPLINE IS   155
    THE ANSWER
    Mercedes Arzu Wilson

24 NEW SOCIAL POLICIES ARE NEEDED 161
National Research Council

CHAPTER 5 ADOLESCENT PREGNANCY IN DEVELOPED NATIONS

25 TEEN PREGNANCY IN WEALTHY NATIONS: 172
THE POINT
Jacqueline Darroch Forrest
26 TEEN PREGNANCY IN WEALTHY NATIONS: 179
THE COUNTERPOINT
Robert G. Marshall
27 TEEN PREGNANCY IN WEALTHY NATIONS: 187
AN ALTERNATIVE PERSPECTIVE
Joy Dryfoos

Appendix 197
Bibliography 202

REASONING SKILL DEVELOPMENT

These activities may be used as individualized study guides for students in libraries and resource centers or as discussion catalysts in small group and classroom discussions.

1 What is Editorial Bias? 57
2 Interpreting Editorial Cartoons 112
3 What is Political Bias? 142
4 Recognizing Author's Point of View 169
5 Examining Counterpoints 195

IDEAS in CONFLICT ®

This series features ideas in conflict on political, social and moral issues. It presents counterpoints, debates, opinions, commentary and analysis for use in libraries and classrooms. Each title in the series uses one or more of the following basic elements:

Introductions that present an issue overview giving historic background and/or a description of the controversy.

Counterpoints and debates carefully chosen from publications, books, and position papers on the political right and left to help librarians and teachers respond to requests that treatment of public issues be fair and balanced.

Symposiums and forums that go beyond debates that can polarize and oversimplify. These present commentary from across the political spectrum that reflect how complex issues attract many shades of opinion.

A global emphasis with foreign perspectives and surveys on various moral questions and political issues that will help readers to place subject matter in a less culture-bound and ethno-centric frame of reference. In an ever shrinking and interdependent world, understanding and cooperation are essential. Many issues are global in nature and can be effectively dealt with only by common efforts and international understanding.

Reasoning skill study guides and discussion activities provide ready made tools for helping with critical reading and evaluation of content. The guides and activities deal with one or more of the following:

RECOGNIZING AUTHOR'S POINT OF VIEW

INTERPRETING EDITORIAL CARTOONS

VALUES IN CONFLICT

WHAT IS EDITORIAL BIAS?

WHAT IS SEX BIAS?
WHAT IS POLITICAL BIAS?
WHAT IS ETHNOCENTRIC BIAS?
WHAT IS RACE BIAS?
WHAT IS RELIGIOUS BIAS?

*From across **the political spectrum** varied sources are presented for research projects and classroom discussions. Diverse opinions in the series come from magazines, newspapers, syndicated columnists, books, political speeches, foreign nations, and position papers by corporations and non-profit institutions.*

About the Editor

Gary E. McCuen is an editor and publisher of anthologies for public libraries and curriculum materials for schools. Over the past 17 years his publications of over 200 titles have specialized in social, moral and political conflict. They include books, pamphlets, cassettes, tabloids, filmstrips and simulation games, many of them designed from his curriculums during 11 years of teaching junior and senior high school social studies. At present he is the editor and publisher of the *Ideas in Conflict* series and the *Editorial Forum* series.

CHAPTER 1

GLOBAL PERSPECTIVES ON ADOLESCENT PREGNANCY

1   U.S. TEEN PREGNANCY RATES ARE FALLING
    Eleanor J. Bader

2   THE RATES ARE RISING
    General Accounting Office

3   ADOLESCENT FERTILITY: WORLDWIDE
    CONCERNS
    Judith Senderowitz and John M. Paxman

4   ADOLESCENT FERTILITY IN NIGERIA
    The Pathfinder Fund

5   TEEN PREGNANCY IN SCOTLAND
    Family Planning Perspectives

6   PREGNANCY RATES IN THE CARIBBEAN
    Tirbani P. Jagdeo

7   TEENAGE SEXUALITY AND PREGNANCY IN
    AUSTRALIA
    Stefania Siedlecky

8   EARLY PREGNANCY IN BRAZIL AND
    GUATEMALA
    Marilyn Edmunds and John M. Paxman

1 GLOBAL PERSPECTIVES ON ADOLESCENT PREGNANCY

U.S. TEEN PREGNANCY RATES ARE FALLING

Eleanor J. Bader

Eleanor J. Bader is a correspondent for the Guardian, *a radical journal of social and political opinion.*

Points to Consider

1. How much money was spent on welfare, food stamps and medical assistance to teen mothers in 1985?
2. What was the nature of the Wisconsin bill dealing with teen pregnancy?
3. What is the "grandparents' liability" clause?
4. How is the role of self-esteem described?
5. Why does society value ignorance?

Eleanor J. Bader, "The Birth Rate Falls," *Guardian,* March 12, 1986, p. 7.

As a society we worship at the altar of sex. It's the payoff. Not everyone can have the goodies, the power, the money, but everyone can have sex and it will be wonderful.

Surprisingly, teen pregnancy rates are falling. In the early 1970s, 61.7 births per 1000 teenagers were recorded. In 1983, the rate was 51.7 per 1000, dropping below 500,000 for the first time since 1960. But the experts are still dismayed: In 1985, $16.6 billion was spent on welfare, food stamps and medical assistance to teen mothers and babies, far too much for an administration hellbent on Gramm-Rudman social service cuts and military increases.

The whole question of teen pregnancy and adolescent sexuality is hot on today's social service agenda. In fact, panic has set in. The panic is couched in inflammatory language: "babies having babies," "moral responsibility," "the value of manhood," and "the weakening moral fiber of the family." For some who attended the annual Children's Defense Fund (CDF) conference Feb. 26–28 in Washington, D.C., the whole gamut of questions creates fertile ground for compromise between right-wing, religious fundamentalist and liberal communities.

"The family is the next big social issue," said Jesse Oliver, a Texas Democrat sitting in that state's legislature. "We need to emphasize morals. When economic issues and obvious moral issues are brought together, there will be an explosion of change. Our job is to take the economic issues and wrap them into the spiritual and moral issues of community." Some 1500 people, at least half of them Black, applauded loudly, shaking their heads in agreement.

The family and notion of familial responsibility for the behavior of its offspring was a favorite theme of this year's "Speakout '86" conference. The audience listened eagerly, carefully, to Marlin Schneider, author of Wisconsin's pioneering "Abortion Prevention and Family Responsibility Law of 1985." The bill was drafted, he said, by 20 people—eight legislators and 12 members of the public—"to reduce the number of abortions by reducing the number of teen pregnancies." According to Schneider, committee members were both pro- and anti-abortion, and included delegates from Planned Parenthood, Wisconsin Citizens Con-

10

Cost of Teen Pregnancies

Teenage childbearing cost the nation $16.6 billion last year, and the 385,000 children who were the firstborn of adolescents in 1985 will receive $6 billion in welfare benefits during the next 20 years, said a study released this week.

The first baby born to a teenager last year will receive $15,620 in welfare payments and other government support by the time the child reaches age 20, according to the study released by the privately financed Center for Population Options.

By the time these babies reach 20, the Government will have spent $6.04 billion to support them through Aid to Families With Dependent Children, Medicaid and food stamps, said the report entitled "Estimates of Public Costs for Teenage Childbearing" . . .

The report said a third of the welfare total, $2.4 billion, could have been saved had teenage mothers waited until they had reached age 20 to have their first baby.

Associated Press, February 20, 1986

cerned for Life, the state Catholic Conference and the Wisconsin Women's Organization.

Grandparents Liable?

The Wisconsin bill has three parts. The first allocates $1 million for adolescent pregnancy prevention and services to pregnant minors. This segment of the bill includes a media campaign mandated to "counter the beautiful people on TV and teach adolescent sexual responsibility." The second section sets up a state adoption center "as an alternative to abortion."

The last and most controversial portion of the bill is a grandparents' liability clause, which forces the parents of a minor to support both the minor and her baby until she is either 18 or able to support the child herself. Likewise, it forces the parents of the adolescent father to provide support. Even married teenagers are governed by this bill; it allows no exemption for emancipated minors. As it is written, if a young woman goes on welfare either while she is pregnant or after, she is required to sue her parents or guardians in order to qualify for benefits. As if this were not enough, she also has to institute a paternity case if the identity of the father is in question. If it is not, she has to sue the man's parents for support. Once such litigation is initiated, the baby and its mother can get benefits, pending court resolution.

"Snarlin' Marlin," as his constituents have dubbed him, has no idea how much money this type of bill will save the state, nor does he know how many young people will be affected by it. His only care, he said, was "shifting family responsibility back to the family."

Syndicated columnist Ellen Goodman said it best: "The average 14- or 15-year-old is biologically an adult. He doesn't need a parent's permission to have sex. She can get pregnant despite a family's veto. No parent can legally force a daughter, let alone a daughter-in-law, to have an abortion. Yet that same parent can be forced to pay for the grandchild until son or daughter is 18. The law to foster family communication may turn into a battlefield between the Hatfields and the McCoys."

Reality notwithstanding, this "innovative approach" has been picked up by other states and is currently pending in Connecticut, Arkansas, Texas and Maryland. The impact of Wisconsin's law, both in terms of dollars and lives, will be studied in 1988; findings must be submitted to the state legislature before January 1, 1989, for evaluation.

Self-Esteem

Another dominant theme at the CDF conference was building self-esteem and the belief in a bright future. That 41.9% of Black and 27.3% of Latino teens are officially unemployed did not daunt the speakers. Atlanta Mayor Andrew Young, for one, still thinks that "there is a future out there if they can apply themselves, discipline themselves. There are rewards for self-discipline and study."

Ignore, for a moment, that in 1975, 8 million young people were employed where there are only 6.3 million youths employed today. Ignore that in 1980 there were 1 million federally-funded summer jobs, while today there are fewer than 750,000. And ignore the fact that cuts in Pell grants to low-income college students will prevent 700,000 young people from getting financial aid in fiscal 1987. Furthermore, ignore the fact that those students who do go to college will face a 60% reduction in college work study grants.

"I am the eternal optimist," said Andre Watson of Washington, D.C.'s Concerned Black Men. "These problems can be transcended, overcome. You, the individual has this power. The power of positivity."

"It smacks of the old 'you can pull yourself up by your bootstraps' thinking and ignores the realities of racism, sexism and classism and symptoms like nutritional deprivation, overcrowded housing, illiteracy, bad schools and just plain personal pain," said Iris, a social worker from South Carolina. "All it does is tell the kid it's his or her own fault they're having trouble making it." But Iris was in the minority at the conference. The mood was optimistic, almost jubilant, in its belief that that pie is big enough to go around and all who are hungry can come and eat.

As to teenage pregnancy itself, it is bad, says CDF literature, because "it interrupts and often forestalls the adolescent's transition to adulthood. Adolescent parenthood is a problem because it often precedes the completion of education, securing of employment and the creation of a stable relationship, and because it makes the completion of these transitional steps very difficult." . . .

That many teens are ignorant about sexual issues is clear, as is the need for quality, explicit sex education. Robert Johnson, a New Jersey physician, hammered this home with the story of a teenage couple who got birth control pills and alternated taking them, the man one month, the woman the next, so that they could share the responsibility. Stories of teens who believed they couldn't get pregnant the first time are well-known, as is the fact that most adolescents wait 9–12 months after becoming heterosexually active before going for birth control. They go then due to their own, or a friend's, pregnancy scare, say experts.

Ignorance Valued

According to Joanne Rocco Bruno, director of education for Planned Parenthood of Eastern Pennsylvania, "Most teens who engage in sex report that they are in a strong, committed, caring relationship. They report that they enjoy intercourse." But 45% of

2500 young people surveyed, she said, could not answer questions about contraceptives and 60% used nothing the first time they had intercourse.

"As a society we worship at the altar of sex," Bruno said. "It's the payoff. Not everyone can have the goodies, the power, the money, but everyone can have sex and it will be wonderful. This is the message—seduction, then prohibition. Sex is romantic, exciting, but good girls say no." The fear, she said, is that knowledge leads to experimentation. "Sexuality is the one area in which we value ignorance," she concluded.

The fact that interest in teen sexuality is linked with an interest in preventing teen pregnancy, at a time when the pregnancy rate is falling on its own, raises many questions. Why, for example, are foundations and corporations funding these programs in amounts that rival expenditures on services for the homeless, but not housing? Gaye Williams, vice chair of the National Political Caucus of Black Women, had a guess. "Young Black people are being set up to take the blame for the destruction of the welfare system," she said. "The Reagan administration has had on its agenda getting rid of welfare since 1980. But how can they accomplish that without looking mean, cruel and uncaring? So they push the image of young, oversexed, irresponsible Black men with Black girls who only want to lay back and have babies. The message is that welfare leads to the breakdown of the family and if we didn't have this evil welfare system they'd be productive members of society."

That any 1500 adults in one place at one time can formulate the solution to adolescent problems is, in and of itself, unlikely. Williams called for the input of teen boys and girls in all programs dealing with teen sexuality.

Programs for sex education, contraception and abortion must be made widely available. At the same time, facing today's reality, why shouldn't teen pregnancy be an option, with school-based childcare, school-based contraceptive dispensaries, counseling and the building of adequate housing, health care facilities, nutritional programs and job training programs? Why not build in supports instead of setting up barriers that virtually insure young women and their babies a life of poverty? These are the questions the progressive community needs to be asking. At the same time it needs to push mainstream social service providers to reject a profamily position that out-right-wings the right wing.

2 GLOBAL PERSPECTIVES ON ADOLESCENT PREGNANCY

THE RATES ARE RISING

General Accounting Office

The following comments were taken from a report by the General Accounting Office titled Teenage Pregnancy: 500,000 Births a Year But Few Tested Programs.

Points to Consider

1. What is known about the extent of teenage pregnancy?
2. What has happened to the pregnancy rates and the birth rates?
3. How are teenage pregnancy and poverty related?
4. What risks are associated with teenage pregnancy?
5. What programs are available to help prevent teen pregnancy?
6. How is the federal government involved in local efforts to prevent teen pregnancy?

Teenage Pregnancy, U.S. General Accounting Office, July, 1986, pp. 8–15.

Compared to women who delay their childbearing, women who bear children before the age of 18 generally experience more birth complications and show deficits in educational attainment and income.

In 1983, there were 500,000 live births and more than 1 million pregnancies in the United States to women younger than 20. While teenage pregnancy rates increased during the past decade, teenage birthrates, overall, declined. Although reliable information is not available on the extent of teenage pregnancy and births among the poor, it is known that birthrates are increasing for unmarried teenagers and have barely declined for very young teenagers—two groups at particular risk of negative health, educational, and social outcomes. Additionally, the number of births to unmarried teenagers varies dramatically by state of residence.

Teenage Pregnancy Rates Have Increased While Birthrates Have Declined Overall

Combining data from surveys of health care providers with federal natality statistics to include births, abortions, and miscarriages, the Alan Guttmacher Institute has estimated that teenage pregnancy rates have increased (see figure 1).

—In 1972 (the first year for which data are available), about 95 in every 1,000 women 15 to 19 years old became pregnant;
—In 1981 (the year of the most recent data), the rate was estimated at about 111 in 1,000.

Teenage birthrates, however, have declined, mirroring the decline in birthrates for all women.

—In 1952, the overall birthrate was 86 in 1,000 among women 15 to 19 years old;
—in 1972, the rate was 62 in 1,000; and
—in 1982, the rate was 53 in 1,000. (In 1983, the year of the most recent data, the rate was 52 in 1,000).

Increased abortion rates for teenagers are believed to account for most of the differences in the pregnancy and birth trends.

Figure 1: Adolescent Pregnancy Rates and Outcomes in the United States in 1970-81 [a]

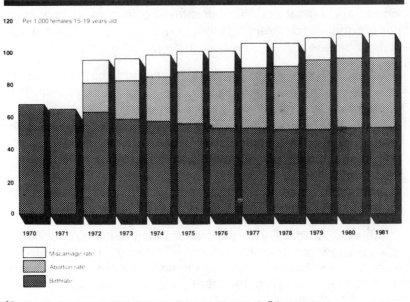

120   Per 1 000 females 15-19 years old

Miscarriage rate
Abortion rate
Birthrate

[a] The pregnancy rate is the sum of the birthrate, abortion rate, and miscarriage rate. Data on pregnancy, abortion, and miscarriage are not available before 1972, because abortion was not legal in many areas before 1972

Source Adapted from U S House of Representatives, Select Committee on Children, Youth, and Families, *Teenage Pregnancy: What Is Being Done? A State-by-State Look* (Washington, D C, U S Government Printing Office, January 1986), p 20, fig 1 The data on pregnancy and abortion are unpublished data from the Alan Guttmacher Institute

Limited Information Is Available on the Extent of Teenage Pregnancy Among the Poor

Compared to women who delay their childbearing, women who bear children before the age of 18 generally experience more birth complications and show deficits in educational attainment and income. Their children have been found to have a higher risk of congenital defects, childhood disease, and developmental lags than children of mothers in their twenties. Teenage childbearing in the context of poverty is believed to increase the probability of these negative consequences and to require additional health and social services to avert these consequences.

To estimate the extent of teenage pregnancy among the poor—and, thus, the need for additional services—we investi-

17

gated nine government and private data bases on fertility, income, and teenagers. We found that no reliable estimates of poor pregnant and parenting teenagers are readily available, for a variety of reasons:

—mothers' income information is not included in birth records,
—household income information is not accurately reported in surveys of teenagers,
—government fertility surveys have excluded teenagers younger than 18 from their samples, and
—the standard national survey of household income reports the number of families with income below the poverty level but excludes from its count families headed by teenagers (or others) that reside in larger households.

Therefore, to identify the populations most in need of services, we examined the available data on other characteristics of teenage births that research has identified as being associated with negative outcomes for teenage pregnancy: age, marital status, and education.

Increasing Proportions of Pregnant and Parenting Teenagers Are at Risk of Negative Outcomes

Although birthrates have declined for teenagers as a whole, they have not declined for some who are at particularly high risk of the negative consequences of childbearing.

—The rate for older teenagers (18 to 19) decreased dramatically after 1970, but the rate for younger teenagers (15 to 17) did not decrease as much.
—The birthrate for very young teenagers (younger than 15) barely declined at all; 1.2 in 1,000 gave birth in 1972, and in 1982, the rate was 1.1 in 1,000.
—The rate for unmarried teenagers (15 to 19) rose from 23 in 1,000 in 1972 to 29 in 1,000 in 1982, resulting in 270,000 births (30 in 1,000) in 1983.
—It appears that not only are younger mothers less likely to have married or completed high school by the time of a birth but that also the younger the mother, the less likely she is to have completed school by the time she reaches her twenties (see table 1).

Table 1

**1983 High School Status
of Women Ages 20–26 Who Were Teenage Mothers**

Age at first birth	Dropout	Received diploma	Received general equivalency diploma
Younger than 15	70%	23%	6%
15	55	24	21
16	51	28	21
17	47	38	15
18	38	52	10
19	23	68	9
At least 20	10	86	4

Percentages do not add to 100 because of rounding.

Source: F. L. Mott and W. Marsiglio, "Early Childbearing and Completion of High School," *Family Planning Perspectives*, 17:5 (1985), 236, table 3.

Current Approaches and Proposals for Addressing Teenage Pregnancy

Communities across the nation currently offer a broad range of programs addressing teenage pregnancy. The programs generally attempt either to prevent unintended teenage pregnancy or to provide services to assist pregnant teenagers and teenage mothers in preventing some of the negative consequences for mother and child. The federal role appears limited at present to a single demonstration program aimed solely at these activities and nine other grant programs that provide services relevant to teenage pregnancy for the general population. The legislative proposals by Senator Chafee and Senator Moynihan would create new grant programs to expand services targeted exclusively to pregnant and parenting young women.

Existing Programs Describe a Wide Variety of Approaches

Reviews of the program literature, which include surveys of state and local government agencies, have uncovered a wide variety of approaches to preventing pregnancy and providing assistance to teenagers who are pregnant or mothers. Although some local sponsors provide both prevention and assistance services, we have separated these two program types, for convenience. Projects frequently resemble hybrids. We found the five types of prevention programs and five types of service programs that we list in table 2 below and table 3.

Table 2

**Services Provided in Five Reported Types
of Pregnancy Prevention Programs**

Program type	Typically included	Possibly included
Sexuality education	Class instruction in puberty and reproduction	Discussion of family life, sex roles, interpersonal relationships, or family planning
Interpersonal values discussion	Outreach workshops and seminars on peer pressure, interpersonal relationships, and family communication	Assertiveness training, education for self-esteem, or ongoing peer support groups
Parents as educators programs	Outreach workshops and seminars on adolescent development, peer pressure, and family communication	Sexuality education materials provided to teenagers
Family planning clinics	Physical exams, contraceptive information and supplies, and pregnancy testing and counseling	Community education and outreach or special education and counseling for teenagers or their parents
Comprehensive teenage health clinics	Routine health care, physical exams, health education, and counseling	Substance abuse programs, contraceptive services, or prenatal health care

The Current Federal Role Is Limited

The size of the federal government's role in the variety of existing programs is not precisely known but appears limited. While several federal grant programs are relevant to teenage pregnancy programs, information on the number of pregnant and parenting teenagers who are served and on the amount of federal funds spent on this subpopulation is available at the federal level for only one of these programs.

20

Prevention Programs

*"Reducing prevention programs will in effect in-
crease the number of families which must rely on public
assistance,"* concluded a study by the Washington-
based Center for Population Options.

The study found that a teenager who bears a child
will cost taxpayers $15,620 by the time the child is 20.
If teenage girls wait until they are 20—when they would
have better job prospects—before having a baby, the
government would save one-third of the welfare costs,
or $2.4 billion a year.

Boston Globe, February 24, 1986

—Only one program serves teenage mothers exclusively—the
AFL program. Its fiscal year 1986 appropriation was $15 million,
and it funded prevention and service demonstration projects
and research on the antecedents and consequences of the
problem of teenage pregnancy.

—Three grant programs have pregnant and parenting teenagers
as a target group: Family Planning Services (which targets all
teenagers); Employment Training Services for the Disadvantaged, under the Job Training Partnership Act (JTPA); and the
Special Supplemental Food Program for Women, Infants, and
Children (WIC). National information on funds allocated to
teenagers through these programs is not maintained.

—Six programs provide services relevant to poor pregnant and
parenting teenagers: the maternal and child health block grants
and the social services block grants, the program for community health centers, employment services and job training
grants (demonstrations under the JTPA), child welfare grants,
and community services block grants. National information on
funds allocated by these programs to pregnant and parenting
teenagers is not maintained.

Although the expenditures of these programs on teenage
pregnancy are not known, the federal role appears to be
secondary to the local one. A national survey of the 153 largest

U.S. cities in 1979–80 asked local health and education department officials about special programs for pregnant teenagers. Of the 127 responding cities, 90 reported that special programs were provided and that most of these received public funds from one or more sources: 67 percent received local funds, 59 percent received state funds, and 47 percent received federal funds. Neither the amount received nor the share of total funds was reported.

Table 3

Services Provided in Five Reported Types of Postpregnancy Programs

Program type	Typically included	Possibly included
Perinatal health care and parenting education	Medical exams and care; information on pregnancy, childbirth, and infant health care; and nutritional advice and supplements	Family planning services, information on child growth and development, intensive training in mother-child interaction, or social service referrals
Residential care	Residential care for pregnant teenagers, prenatal care and childbirth education, and individual and group counseling	Arrangements to continue education, parenting education, family planning services, or residential services for teenage mothers and their children
Alternative school programs	Academic instruction (at home or in a separate building) and referrals for perinatal health care and parenting education	Family planning services, group counseling, or special childbirth and parenting classes for students remaining in regular classes
Social services with referrals	Outreach, individual or group counseling, and referrals for health and education services	Life-skills training, preparation for general equivalency diploma, or vocational assistance
Comprehensive services	Perinatal health care and parenting education, arrangements to continue education, group counseling, referral and followup using a case-management system	Vocational assistance, family planning services, child care, or single assignments of staff

GLOBAL PERSPECTIVES ON ADOLESCENT PREGNANCY

ADOLESCENT FERTILITY: WORLDWIDE CONCERNS

Judith Senderowitz and John M. Paxman

Childbearing by women under age 20—adolescent fertility—is not a new phenomenon in world history. Historically, marriage has come early in most countries and childbearing was expected to follow soon after. This is still the norm in many developing countries where fertility rates of women under 20, though now declining, are still very high. In developed countries, adolescent fertility rates are much lower and declining in concert with the rates of older women, but there is concern with rising rates of abortion and out-of-wedlock births among teenage women.

What *is* new in the past decade or so is the growing recognition of and concern over the adverse health, social, economic and demographic effects of adolescent fertility. Rates of illness and mortality are significantly higher for teenage mothers and their infants than they are for older mothers. Early initiation of childbearing is likely to mean truncated education, lower future family income, and also larger completed family sizes, which, along with shorter time spans between generations, contribute to rapid population growth. Demographically, the impact of childbearing among women under 20 in developing nations is further heightened by the large numbers and proportions of young people aged 10–19 in these nations, now and in the future, due to past high fertility. Even if fertility rates were to

Judith Senderowitz and John M. Paxman, "Adolescent Fertility: Worldwide Concerns," Population Reference Bureau, Inc., Vol. 40, No. 2, April, 1985.

drop precipitously among adolescent women in developing nations, their sheer numbers mean that their fertility will continue to have a major impact on world population growth for some time to come.

The International Population Conference of August 1984 in Mexico City addressed the issue of teenage pregnancy and childbearing in four of the 88 Recommendations endorsed by delegates of the 147 nations represented at the conference. Government policies are advised to "encourage delay in the commencement of childbearing" and to "raise the age of entry into marriage" (Recommendations 7 and 8). Another recommendation encourages "community education to change prevailing attitudes which countenance pregnancy and childbearing at young ages, recognizing that pregnancy occurring in adolescent girls, whether married or unmarried, has adverse effects on the morbidity and mortality of both mother and child" (Recommendation 18). And a fourth recommendation urges governments "to ensure that adolescents, both boys and girls, receive adequate education, including family-life and sex education . . . and suitable family planning information and services" (Recommendation 29).

The designation by the United Nations of 1985 as International Youth Year is an added incentive to focus on the dimensions and problems of adolescent fertility as among the important issues to be addressed in the Year's objective of improving the world situation of youth. Toward that end, this *Bulletin* explores the following questions. What are the current and projected numbers of adolescents worldwide? What are the patterns of their fertility-related behavior: premarital sexual intercourse, age at marriage and first birth, and levels of fertility, contraceptive use, and abortion practice? How do laws and policies help or hinder efforts to meet the reproductive health needs of adolescents? And what programs are being mounted worldwide to address the implications of all this?

We begin with defining adolescence.

Definition of Adolescence

Adolescence is said to be the process through which an individual makes the transition from childhood to adulthood. Most cultures relate the beginning of this process to the onset of

Soviet Sexual Ignorance

Widespread "sexual illiteracy" among the people and doctors of the Soviet Union has led to a high rate of abortion and divorce, a leading sociologist said in an unusually explicit article on sex . . .

Igor Kon, an author and doctor of philosophy, noted that there is no sex education in Soviet schools, few trained sex counselors and virtually no books available on the subject. To make matters worse, he said, most parents are reluctant to talk about sex with their doctors or children.

Associated Press, July 6, 1987

puberty, but differ widely over when it ends, as described by James Chui: "In many developing countries, especially in rural and underdeveloped areas, a girl is often considered to be an adult at the time when menstruation is established regularly. They tend to marry early and do not go to school. The transition from childhood to adulthood in such cases is quick, and the notion of adolescence does not exist. On the other hand, in developed countries and increasingly in urban areas of developing countries where rapid social changes are taking place with modernization, young people go to school and tend to marry late. There is a long transition from childhood to adulthood, and the notion of adolescence emerges. There is thus a continuum between quick and slow transition in different societies."

These variations make it difficult to define adolescence in specific universal terms. But in dealing with the issue of early childbearing, it is most useful to adopt the age limits of 10–20 suggested by a World Health Organization Committee on the Health Problems of Adolescence. To pinpoint the problems, where data are available, social scientists and medical researchers often prefer to distinguish early adolescence (ages 10–14) from late adolescence (ages 15–19) . . .

The increase in numbers of adolescents and the patterns of their fertility-related behavior vary widely between the developing and developed regions, between countries within these regions, and between urban and rural areas and different cultures within countries.

Numbers of Adolescents

According to the "medium variant" of assessments prepared in 1982 by the United Nations, there are just over a billion young people aged 10–19 in the world in 1985—526 million boys and 506 million girls. Eighty-three percent of these adolescents live in the developing countries, where they make up 23 percent of the total population (see Figure 1). In the developed countries as a whole, adolescents comprise 15 percent of the total population. By 2020, according to the U.N. medium projections, the world total of adolescents aged 10–19 will be over 1.3 billion, an increase of 27 percent in 35 years. Of these, 1.1 billion, or 86 percent, will live in the developing nations of Africa, Asia (minus Japan), and Latin America . . .

Fertility

Rates and levels of adolescent fertility, largely reflecting marriage patterns, also vary widely both between and within the developing and the developed worlds. Worldwide, age-specific fertility rates for women aged 15–19 range from as low as 4 births per 1,000 in Japan and 9 in the Netherlands in 1981 to 253 in Bangladesh in 1976 and 302 in Mauritania in 1981. The rates of the developing nations are generally extremely high relative to the developed world. In sub-Saharan Africa virtually all the rates are well over 100. In Latin America, they are more moderate, with most in the low 100s or below. And the developing nations of Asia again display the greatest variation, from several, like Bangladesh, with rates far above 100, down to countries with rates far below the 53 of the U.S. in 1982, such as China (15 in 1981), South Korea (11 in 1974), and Singapore (12 in 1981).

Although the rates are collectively lowest in developed nations, in some, as in the U.S., they are relative high: Greece (53), Italy (51), Portugal (41), and again in Eastern European countries, Bulgaria (81), Czechoslovakia (49), Hungary (63), Romania (72), and Yugoslavia (49). In the U.S. in 1982, while the overall fertility rate for 15–19 year olds was 53 births per 1,000 women, it varied from 45 for white women to 97 for black women . . .

Figure 1. Adolescents Aged 10-19 in the Population Age Pyramids of Developing and Developed Countries: 1985, 2020

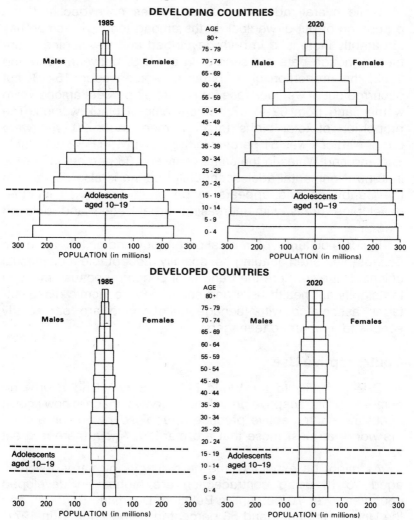

Source: United Nations, *World Population Prospects as Assessed in 1982*, medium variant, forthcoming.

Note: Developing countries = Africa, Asia (minus Japan), Latin America, and Oceania (minus Australia and New Zealand).
Developed countries = Europe, Canada, United States, U.S.S.R., Japan, Australia, New Zealand.

27

Out-of-Wedlock Childbearing

While overall adolescent fertility rates have declined, the proportion of out-of-wedlock births among teenage women has apparently increased in both developed and developing countries, although data are scarce. In the U.S. between 1970 and 1982, the proportion of all births to women aged 15–19 that occurred out of wedlock rose from 17 to 37 percent among white women and from 62 to 87 percent among black women. The proportion of total births to all women under 20 that were out-of-wedlock was 51 percent in the U.S. in 1982, 52 percent in England and Wales in the same year, and 38 percent in France in 1980. Nonmarital adolescent childbearing is also common in the Caribbean and appears to be on the increase in other developing areas with increasing urbanization and delayed marriage.

In some cultures, premarital pregnancy and childbearing are acceptable, often leading to socially acceptable consensual unions. But elsewhere the trend is of concern because many of the significant health risks and social and economic disadvantages associated with teenage childbearing are particularly serious for unmarried teenagers.

Contraceptive Use

Due primarily to the World Fertility Survey and a growing number of contraceptive prevalence surveys, much is now known about the contraceptive practice of adolescent women around the world, at least those that are married. Again there is great variety.

As might be expected, the percentages of married women aged 15–19 using contraception are highest in developed countries: over 70 percent in Belgium, Denmark, Portugal, and the United Kingdom, and 53 percent in both Hungary (in 1977) and the U.S. (in 1982). On average the proportions are lowest in Africa, where the concept of family planning, at least for limiting fertility, has yet to be fully accepted . . .

What little is known about contraceptive use among unmarried teenagers who are sexually active, again mostly from often small surveys in developed countries, indicates that their contraceptive behavior is inconsistent at best and often ineffective . . .

Many factors explain these behavior patterns: inaccurate knowledge about the reproductive process and contraception, inaccessibility of services, personal, peer group and social pressures, adolescents' tendency not to plan ahead, etc. . . .

Abortion

Among the most dramatic reflections of premarital sexual activity among adolescents are figures on abortion. Available data indicate that unmarried women account for the majority of abortions in most countries, whether legal or illegal, and many of these are teenagers.

Abortions obtained by women under 20 make up a substantial proportion of total abortions in the countries, mostly in the developed world, where the procedure is legal and widely available . . .

Rates for teenage women in countries where abortion is legal rose steadily during the 1970s and only recently have begun to level off or decline . . .

Causes of Adolescent Fertility

One biological factor common to earlier sexual activity and pregnancy is the reduced age at menarche (onset of first menstruation) reported in cultures as diverse as those in Africa, Asia and Europe . . . Menarche both renders a woman's body capable of conception and predisposes the individual to become sexually receptive . . .

Changing Societal Values

In Africa, for example, traditional systems of preparation for adult life are being threatened, resulting in the loss of parental and community guidance in the area of sexuality. At the same time, aspects of urbanization, such as housing shortages and increased education for females, create an environment for increased interaction between adolescent males and females and allow for peer pressure to exert its powerful force. These influences of permissiveness and increased opportunity for sexual expression, however, must be viewed in the light of traditional values which are still strong and operating in the same direction. Most African societies place high value on large families, with expectations of early marriage and prompt child-bearing within those marriages.

Other societies where marriage traditionally comes early have been influenced by modern needs and realities to raise the legal age of marriage. In India the legal age of marriage is now 18 for women, but many women continue to be married earlier, reflecting the strong pull of traditional values. Religious norms significantly influence adolescent sexual behavior, so that sexual intercourse outside of marriage is generally prohibited by law and condemned by the public, as in Indonesia. However, even in Indonesia shifts are now observable in the big cities.

Many countries are experiencing a real flux in values. Sociologist Mounir Khoury describes Lebanese society as close to "normlessness," with little support for often contradictory norms and values and consequently less direction for adolescents in their sexual behavior. Cuba is an example of a country which underwent significant changes in social mores following its 1959 revolution. Emphasis is placed on involvement of the young, men and women, away from traditional parental control and sexual expectations. No longer does the taboo against premarital sex prevent out-of-wedlock pregnancies. The same diminution of parental and social control is evident in many other societies of Latin America, North America and Europe. These societies have witnessed a long-term evolution of freer sexual expression in general and, in particular, greater independence of young people to participate in these changes.

A major purveyor of the altered values and mores is mass media which increasingly reaches most areas of most countries. Adolescents are avid consumers of the media and are heavily influenced by it. Teenagers in the U.S., for example, watch or listen to major forms of media (television, radio, motion pictures) 45 hours per week, on average. TV in particular seems to communicate a fantasy view of the world in which sex occurs without responsibility and various events (divorces, out-of-wedlock births, abortions) are out of proportion to reality. A dramatic example of changing attitudes is TV reference to sexual intercourse: extramarital sex occurs six times more than sex between spouses and 94 percent of sexual encounters on "soap operas" are between unmarried people . . .

Social and Economic Factors

Many social and economic factors are significant predictors of early sexual activity. In general, the lower the income and education of the parents and the adolescent, the earlier sexual activity begins and the greater the likelihood of an early pregnancy. Family size and structure are also related. The larger the adolescent female's immediate family, the more likely she is to begin sexual activity and childbearing at an early age. In U.S. and Costa Rican studies, a single-parent home increases the chances of sexual activity; where the father is present, his educational level has a negative effect on the probability of intercourse. . . .

Conclusion

Adolescent fertility is perceived and addressed differently in various parts of the world. Thus, attempts to affect it or ameliorate its negative consequences must vary according to cultural realities.

Some cautious generalizations can be made about three distinct, current patterns. The *first,* common in the developing world, is characterized by early age at marriage or consensual union and early and frequent childbearing. Cultural values, especially in Asia, prohibit premarital sexual activity and premarital pregnancy is infrequent or likely to lead to socially sanctioned consensual unions, as in Latin America and evidently in parts of sub-Saharan Africa. Contraceptive use is low, but slowly rising. When abortion is sought, usually by young unmarried girls, it is usually illegal, hence clandestine and potentially dangerous.

The *second,* perhaps polar opposite pattern, exists primarily in developed countries. It is characterized by the onset of sexual experience, often out of wedlock, in the mid- to late teens. Though contraceptives are available, their use is low among unmarried sexually active teenagers, except in some Western European countries, and there is a high incidence of unintended nonmarital pregnancy, significant recourse to abortion (largely legal and safe), late age at marriage, and very low fertility.

The *third* is a middle ground of changing patterns prompted largely by socioeconomic development. With rapid growth of large cities, typical of sub-Saharan Africa, for example, women's economic and employment opportunities are expanding, and age at marriage and first birth is being delayed. The traditional restraints of the first pattern are still evident but less controlling, and, following the second pattern, premarital sexual activity and pregnancy are increasing, as is recourse to abortion. However, overall fertility is beginning to decline as contraception is used more and more, except so far in sub-Saharan Africa.

GLOBAL PERSPECTIVES ON ADOLESCENT PREGNANCY

ADOLESCENT FERTILITY IN NIGERIA

The Pathfinder Fund

Adolescence is a critical period of biological and psychological change. For the 18 million youth in Africa's most populous country, the biological change is liable to coincide with social transitions and stresses. Nigeria's youth are sexually active. Fertility is high among young Nigerian women, who typically marry at very early ages. Among unmarried adolescents, unwanted pregnancies are a common problem. Because of their high rate of sexual activity and rapidly growing numbers, Nigeria's youth population is becoming increasingly critical to the formulation of health and social policies.

This executive Summary will survey three areas of particular concern:

● The increased health risks and social disadvantages facing adolescent mothers and their children.

● The growing epidemic of abortions caused by unwanted pregnancies, particularly among the unmarried.

● The high incidence of sexually transmitted diseases (STDs) among young people, a leading cause of future infertility.

Demographic Profile of Youth

● The 18 million youth aged 15–24 comprise 19 percent of Nigeria's total population.

The Pathfinder Fund, "Adolescent Fertility in Nigeria, 1986."

- This group is growing at a faster rate than the overall population. Its numbers are projected to almost double in size, to 31 million people, by the year 2000.
- Forty-four percent of women aged 15–19 are already married.
- In the 20–24 age group, 85 percent of women have been married and nearly a third have had three or more children.
- A recent Ibadan survey of unmarried adolescents aged 14–25 shows that half the girls and nearly four-fifths of the boys have had sexual relations by the time they are 18 years old.

The High Percentage of Adolescent Births

- Young women will continue to account for a high proportion of Nigeria's total fertility. Almost half of the country's women of childbearing age are 15 to 24 years old. Improvements in health conditions have resulted in a steady decline in the age of menarche (bringing earlier sexual maturity) and reduced adolescent subfecundity. Because women continue to marry very young, there is a dramatic impact on Nigeria's birthrate from these combined factors.
- While significant family pressure is still exerted on couples to bear children during the first year of marriage, traditional methods of birth regulation are declining. As young wives become more urbanized and better educated, they are generally less inclined to undergo long periods of sexual abstinence in order to space births.
- Meanwhile, the use of modern contraceptives, although increasing, is still very low. Only 7 percent of married women in the 20–24 age group, and 4 percent of those aged 15–19, are currently using any form of contraception.

Premarital Pregnancy

- While traditional cultural practices encouraged chastity before marriage, there now appears to be a movement toward sexual permissiveness brought about by urbanization and other social changes which have altered the scope of the adolescent pregnancy problem.
- The limited survey data available show that sexual activity among unwed males and females, particularly in urban areas, is becoming increasingly common. Large numbers of adolescents engage in sexual relations, with many starting as early as age 15

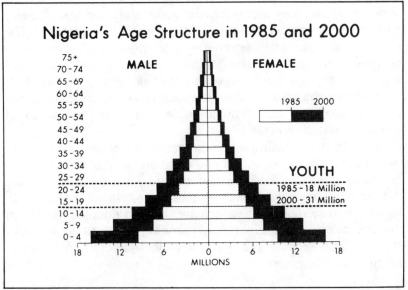

Nigeria's Age Structure in 1985 and 2000

MALE   FEMALE

1985   2000

YOUTH
1985 - 18 Million
2000 - 31 Million

75+
70 - 74
65 - 69
60 - 64
55 - 59
50 - 54
45 - 49
40 - 44
35 - 39
30 - 34
25 - 29
20 - 24
15 - 19
10 - 14
5 - 9
0 - 4

18   12   6   0   6   12   18
MILLIONS

Source: United Nations, 1982 Assessment.

or younger, when access to contraceptive services or even counselling is virtually nonexistent.

● Pregnancies are not isolated cases within the unmarried adolescent population, but are a problem of widespread proportions. According to the 1981–82 Ibadan survey, for example, almost half the sexually active young women interviewed have had at least one pregnancy.

● There is evidence that substantial numbers of pregnancies occur among teenagers during the years of secondary school. One study showed that 55 percent of secondary school girls in Benin City first had sexual intercourse before age 16.

Family Planning for Adolescents

Lack of knowledge and failure to use modern contraception is a major factor contributing to adolescent pregnancies.

● Despite the high rate of adolescent sexual activity, the practice of contraception is not widespread, particularly among secondary school students. Only 8 percent of women aged 15–19 have ever used any method of contraception. Even those who have been pregnant before appear to be lazy about using contraceptives.

• While some young people do know about contraceptives, their information is often incorrect and their attitudes about using contraceptives are often ambivalent or negatively prejudiced. The mortality and morbidity associated with induced abortion are a far greater threat than complications associated with the use of any contraceptive, but adolescents frequently hold the view that contraception is harmful. Many contraceptives, such as condoms and spermicides, also provide protection from the spread of sexually transmitted diseases.

• Despite the government's pronouncement in its 1980–85 development plan that it "will pay more attention to the provision of family planning facilities and ensure that the services are available to those who wish to use them," family planning in Nigeria is only geared toward older married couples. Although the need for adolescent family planning services is acute in Nigeria, adolescents are generally not selected for special programs or treatment.

Health Risks of Early Pregnancy

• Maternity-related complications are among the leading causes of death for women aged 15–24 in Africa, especially in the younger ages. Young women under the age of 18 are 1.5 to 2 times more likely than older women to die due to pregnancy-related causes.

• The medical risks associated with early pregnancy include anemia, bleeding, toxemia, prolonged and difficult labor and urinary and bowel complications. Physical maturity, particularly of the pelvis, often lags behind the ability to conceive. Pregnancy occurring before full reproductive maturity frequently compromises the adolescent's future fertility.

• Early pregnancy poses special health risks not only for the mother but also for the child. The infants of teenagers suffer higher mortality than those of older mothers. They also have higher rates of premature birth and low birth weight. These conditions frequently contribute to long-term mental and physical handicaps.

• While the risks of early pregnancy are lessened by good health care, the bulk of Nigerian adolescents who become pregnant do not receive adequate medical attention. Perhaps because of ignorance or immaturity, most hesitate a long time before seeing health care personnel, thereby increasing their risk of developing complications.

● The medical risks of pregnancy are aggravated for unmarried adolescents who must contend with social disapproval and who may receive little emotional or familial support during pregnancy. These women are more likely than married women to lose their babies.

Social Consequences of Early Pregnancy

● Early childbearing is strongly associated in research findings with lower social and occupational mobility for both the adolescent parent and the child. Invariably, there is at least a temporary and usually a permanent halt to education. Career opportunities are often cut off and young persons forced into premature marriages or forced to bear children outside marriage.

● Yet, the traditional criteria for acquiring higher social status and prestige are changing, and the role of formal education and a formal sector occupation are replacing the traditional importance of lineage, age, sex and fertility. Thus adolescents have a keen interest in avoiding any interruption which would jeopardize future social and economic prospects.

● Furthermore, the influence of the extended family system (which used to provide for the needs of all children, including those born out of wedlock) is declining, particularly in poor urban areas. Unwanted adolescent pregnancies contribute to the increasing number of neglected and abandoned children in Nigeria.

The Abortion Epidemic

● The upsurge of interest in pursuing higher education and jobs, coupled with more permissive adolescent lifestyles, has contributed to the growing problem of illegal abortion in Nigeria. Despite the risks, abortion is the one course of action chosen by many unmarried pregnant adolescents.

● Nigeria has no nationwide data on abortions, which are illegal except to save the life of the pregnant woman. However, available information from clinics, hospitals and sample surveys demonstrates that the number of abortions is increasing.

- Of all the young unmarried women in the Ibadan survey who became pregnant, 9 out of every 10 had an abortion, including virtually all the university and polytechnic students, and roughly 4 out of 5 secondary school students and working women. Other studies confirm that adolescent abortion is a widespread problem.
- Illegal abortion is one of the main causes of death among unmarried Nigerian women aged 15–24, especially those attending secondary school. Besides the risk of death, clandestine abortions often result in the permanent loss of fertility. For a society in which childbearing is so highly valued this carries with it severe social stigmas.
- Illegal adolescent abortions are seldom performed by qualified doctors. These abortions have high rates of mortality and complications because they usually involve dangerous methods used by incompetent practitioners under poor hygienic conditions. Young women tend to go to a hospital only after life-threatening complications develop.
- In addition to causing human suffering and ill health, clandestine adolescent abortions put a severe strain on hospital resources. The resources diverted for the treatment of illegal abortion complications have not been fully estimated. However, it has been shown over the years that 14 to 25 percent of hospital services have to be committed to the treatment of abortion complications. The average time spent by adolescents with induced abortions at Benin University Teaching Hospital, for example, is 11 days, with stays ranging from 3 to 84 days.

The Spread of Sexually Transmitted Diseases

- The more liberal lifestyles of today's youth enhance the spread of sexually transmitted diseases (STDs). The most common way these diseases are spread is through casual sexual encounters (rather than through contact with prostitutes, as commonly thought).
- Clinic studies demonstrate that adolescents (mainly males) account for well over 30 percent of STD cases.
- STDs are a significant cause of pregnancy wastage and infertility in both men and women. They create individual hardships and are a drain on national resources by depleting funds for health care and contributing to lost productivity.

38

- The diminished sensitivity of STDs to drugs such as penicillin poses a serious threat to the containment of these diseases among both adolescents and the overall population. Another problem is that the majority of those infected, particularly young persons, receive inadequate medical treatment and thus continue to spread the infection.

5 GLOBAL PERSPECTIVES ON ADOLESCENT PREGNANCY

TEEN PREGNANCY IN SCOTLAND

Family Planning Perspectives

Premarital Sexual Intercourse Far More Common Among Scottish Teens Today Than 20 Years Ago

Today's Scottish teenagers are much more likely to engage in premarital intercourse than were adolescents two or three decades ago, although they remain less likely to do so than are their English or Welsh counterparts. According to the results of a recent survey, only six percent of Scottish women born between 1926 and 1930 had premarital intercourse while they were teenagers, compared with 50 percent of those born between 1951 and 1955 and 61 percent of the 1961–1965 cohort. In addition, modern teenagers are less likely to marry than were their recent predecessors. Thus, the length of time during which a Scottish teenager is at risk of having a premarital conception has increased recently. Nevertheless, the probability that Scottish teenagers will become pregnant premaritally appears to have fallen, most likely as a result of high levels of contraceptive use among those who are sexually active.

The Survey

The survey was conducted by the Office of Population Censuses and Surveys, on behalf of the Scottish Home and

Reproduced with permission from *Family Planning Perspectives,* Vol. 18, Number 5, Sept./Oct. 1986.

Health Department, in 1985. A total of 3,400 women aged 16–54 were selected randomly and interviewed concerning their experience of premarital sexual intercourse, conception and contraceptive use as teenagers.

Overall, in each year of the 1950s, about 2–3 percent of unmarried 15–19-year-olds ever had intercourse; in 1964, this proportion was seven percent, and it climbed to over 20 percent in 1981. (Overall levels of premarital teenage sexual experience are lower in Scotland than in Great Britain as a whole: For example, in 1976, 37 percent of all unmarried British teenagers had had intercourse, compared with only 17 percent of single Scottish teenagers.)

An analysis using life tables to determine cohort levels of sexual experience indicates that 50 percent of women born between 1951 and 1955 had premarital intercourse during adolescence, as did 61 percent of women born in the period 1961–1965. However, the author of the survey report comments, despite claims that teenage sexual activity increased only after family planning services became available to single women (in 1968), and especially after such services were made available free of charge through the National Health Service (in 1975), "there were striking increases in teenage intercourse among single girls long before the development of the family planning services and even before the pill became available." For example, she points out that the proportion of young single women who ever had intercourse jumped from six percent of those born between 1926 and 1930 to 16 percent of those born between 1931 and 1935, and to 23 percent of those born in the period 1941–1945.

Until the mid-1950s, the increases in teenage sexual activity were accompanied by increases in the proportion of adolescents who were married. This proportion climbed from 16 percent of women born between 1926 and 1930 to about 29 percent of those born in the period 1941–1950 and 34 percent of those born in 1951–1955. However, among later cohorts, teenage marriage has become less common: Twenty-nine percent of women born in the period 1956–1960 and 22 percent of those born between 1961 and 1965 married as teenagers.

In addition, among women who ever had premarital intercourse as teenagers, anywhere from 33 to 41 percent of those born before 1951 married within nine months of first intercourse.

In contrast, this proportion was only 28 percent among women born between 1951 and 1955, and just 19 percent among those born in the period 1956–1960. The author suggests that when single women became more likely to enter into sexual relationships, in the 1950s and 1960s, "it was often because couples anticipated marriage in the relatively near future. . . . In the later 1960s and [the] 1970s, however, the connection between premarital intercourse and the timing of marriage seems to have become more tenuous."

The Trends

As a result of these trends, the time spent by teenagers at risk of a premarital conception increased substantially in recent years. The author estimates that the median length of time teenagers were at risk of premarital conception rose from around 15 months among women born before 1951 to 27 months for those born between 1956 and 1960. The probability of teenager's having a premarital pregnancy also rose, from six percent among women born in the period 1926–1930 to 21 percent among those born in 1951–1955.

Thereafter, however, the proportion of teenagers conceiving before marriage began to decline, reaching a level of just 10 percent among women born between 1961 and 1965. Thus, the likelihood of premarital pregnancy in the teenage years was almost as low for women born between 1961 and 1965 as it was for those born between 1926 and 1930, even though the latter group was much less likely than the former to have sexual intercourse as adolescents. The investigator points out that the apparent decrease in recent years might have been due to an underreporting of abortions, although a similar trend in premarital conceptions has been observed for England and Wales.

Premarital Pregnancies

The decline in premarital pregnancies in the face of increased sexual activity suggests, therefore, that younger Scottish women have adopted contraception in large numbers. Indeed, the data show that while only 18 percent of the women born between 1946 and 1950 used the pill while they were unmarried teenagers, fully 40 percent of those born in the period 1951–1955 did so. The proportion of women who had unprotected first intercourse while

42

single rose steadily, from five percent of those born between 1926 and 1930 to 25 percent of those born in the period of 1946–1950; however, among later cohorts, the proportion who had unprotected first intercourse remained virtually unchanged, despite the fact that overall rates of adolescent premarital intercourse increased from 36 percent to 61 percent.

At the time of the survey, only three percent of single teenage women who had had intercourse in the previous 12 months had not used some contraceptive method at last intercourse. Indeed, a rising proportion of young women reported that they had obtained a method of birth control prior to first intercourse. Among women born between 1941 and 1945, nine percent reported having been prepared before first intercourse, compared with 36 percent of women born in the period 1951–1955 and 41 percent of those born in 1956–1960.

6 GLOBAL PERSPECTIVES ON ADOLESCENT PREGNANCY

PREGNANCY RATES IN THE CARIBBEAN

Tirbani P. Jagdeo

In 1983, the International Planned Parenthood Federation (IPPF) convened a meeting of international experts in Bellagio, Italy to discuss the situation of youth the world over and to make recommendations for a plan of action that would meet the variegated needs of youth living in diverse socio-cultural and economic settings all over the world.

It was fascinating to see how, in the identification of things young people need, these experts came up with the same set of items—better and expanded educational facilities for the young and, in particular, for young women, expanded and improved employment possibilities, the removal of those socio-cultural fetters that restrain adolescent creativity and their greater participation in the programs and decisions directly impinging upon their lives. Of course, it was recognized that youths in different parts of the world were at different points on the path leading to this enhanced social condition. It was also recognized that the preferred means for getting from one point to another will vary with the cultural ethos of each country. But everywhere it was affirmed that we neglect our youth only at the expense of the future, that we plan for them to the enrichment of the heritage we hope to pass on . . .

Tirbani Jagdeo, "Pregnancy Rates in the Caribbean," Inter-American Parliamentary Group on Population and Development, Barbados, 1985, pp. 2–7.

Teenage Fertility

Why does the problem of teenage fertility loom so large in the thinking of family planning agencies and governments today? Is it because the problem is new? We know for a fact that teenage fertility is not a recent phenomenon—not for Africa nor Asia nor Latin America. It is certainly not new in the Caribbean. For generations, Caribbean women have been producing children in their early years and, on the average, had more children then than their counterparts do today. *The evidence shows that for every Caribbean country adolescent fertility rates were higher thirty years ago than they are today.* Since the fifties, adolescent fertility rates declined steadily in most countries save Dominica, Jamaica, Montserrat and St. Lucia where these rates increased somewhat in the sixties before dipping below the levels observed in 1950.

Complacency

There is, however, little room for complacency. Even in the face of these declines, adolescent fertility rates continue to be in excess of 100 per 1000. This means that on the average, more than one in ten adolescents gives birth to a child every year. Adolescent fertility rates in 1980 were as high as 120 in Guyana, 125 in Grenada, 133 in Jamaica, 143 in St. Kitts-Nevis, 157 in St. Lucia and 164 in St. Vincent. But this is only a partial picture. These figures refer only to live births to teenagers. They do not include various forms of pregnancy wastage due to fetal loss, still-births, and induced and spontaneous abortions. Had all these pregnancies come to term, the fertility rates among our adolescents would have been much higher.

There is one important piece of data that we do not now have. This is the fertility rate among women 17 years old and under. We do have some indirect evidence that fertility rates among this age-group are higher than desirable. We know, for example, that almost 60 per cent of all first births in many Caribbean countries occur to teenagers and that one-half of these are to women 17 years old and under. Data from across the world show that reproductive risks are at a maximum among younger teenagers and that, compared to women in their twenties, they are more likely to suffer from prolonged labor, cervical lacerations, caesarian sections and toxemia. Their babies, also, are more likely to be underweight, small-for-date and premature. In a word, pregnancy among younger teenagers endangers the health of the mother and the child—and this is reason enough to motivate our sustained concern and action with regard to adolescent fertility control.

Human Possibilities

But teenage pregnancy is not simply a matter of numbers and medical consequence. It is also a matter of human possibilities, of life chances. Teenage pregnancy stymies both the personal and social development of young women—a fact that is particularly visible in the area of education. Girls who become pregnant in school seldom ever catch up with those who pass through their school-going years untramelled with the responsibilities and sacrifices of motherhood. This is as true of societies that readmit young mothers into the conventional school system as it is true of societies that do not. In the latter case, the gap between childbearing and non-childbearing teenagers becomes greater and young women end up paying dearly in their later lives for mistakes made when they were still children.

Education

These arguments are particularly pertinent to the Caribbean. Pregnancy is the single most important reason why girls drop out of school. For reasons having to do more with custom than with law, pregnant girls are turned out of school and are seldom ever readmitted into the conventional school system. Many lack the example, the will or the options to pursue educational opportunities beyond what is conventionally available. Since teenage pregnancy in the Caribbean occurs disproportionately among lower income women, these pregnancies serve to trap young women and their children within the stringent social and economic circumstances of their parents.

This is precisely the kind of thing that we cannot afford in the Caribbean. Caribbean leaders and their people have moved far beyond elitist assumptions of growth and have begun to regard access to sound education, good jobs and improved living standards as basic human rights. In the past, people could have

46

related to this matter of limited life chances in terms of the way things always were. Today, they are more likely to see them as a denial of the way things should be. It is a discrepancy that young people have to learn to live with. Some of them lower their expectations of life and settle for less. In settling for less, they give less to society and the quality, drive and motivation of our people suffer. Others, failing to see any resolution of their problems at home, migrate. In fact, over 55 per cent of the natural increase emigrated in the seventies—a figure that supports the feeling that emigration is the single most stabilizing population factor in the Caribbean.

Structural Barrier

These are the considerations that have transformed the *problem* of teenage pregnancy into an *issue* facing individuals, households and nations. We can neither ignore the problem nor diminish its importance. Adolescent fertility undermines what we stand for as a people. It constitutes a powerful structural barrier to the aspirations of our women and the overall development of our societies. When we think of development in the Caribbean and list the problems of capital scarcity, fragile infrastructures and economic diversification, let us also list the constricting consequences of adolescent pregnancy. In doing so, we will be putting people, our young people, at the center of our development strategies. We will be conceiving of development in fundamentally human terms.

GLOBAL PERSPECTIVES ON ADOLESCENT PREGNANCY

TEENAGE SEXUALITY AND PREGNANCY IN AUSTRALIA

Stefania Siedlecky

Society generally has had punitive and judgmental attitudes towards teenage sexuality and pregnancy—directed mainly at girls. There is reluctance to provide adequate sex education for fear of encouraging promiscuity, a reluctance to make contraception more easily available—lest it remove the risk of pregnancy and make sex too easy; if a girl gets pregnant she should not have access to abortion but should continue the pregnancy as the price for her transgression; if she has the baby she should have it adopted to give the child a better chance in life and to help some other woman more deserving than herself; if she keeps the baby she is selfish and irresponsible; if she cannot cope and is forced to later give up the baby she really only wanted a toy to play with—the "baby doll" syndrome. She "goes out and gets herself pregnant" because she is depressed or otherwise disturbed or she wants to draw the supporting parents benefit and be a burden on the taxpayer. There are mis-statements and accusations of increasing sexual activity and promiscuity among teenagers and increasing numbers of teenage births. It takes two people to produce a pregnancy but only one has a baby and bears the weight of society's disapproval.

Stefania Siedlecky, "Trends in Teenage Births," Australian Department of Health, 1985, pp. 2–14.

Changing Attitudes

Fortunately, attitudes are changing and many of the myths surrounding teenage sexuality and pregnancy are being dispelled. This paper looks at trends in births and pregnancies among Australian teenagers as a means of exposing some of these myths. It updates previous papers and shows that the decline in teenage pregnancies and births is continuing in Australia.

Data used in this paper have been taken from
1. Australian Bureau of Statistics publications
2. Annual reports of the Committee appointed to examine and report on abortions notified in South Australia 1971–1984 . . .

Trends in Births Among Australian Teenagers

Paradoxically, concern about teenage pregnancy and births has increased at a time when birthrates among Australian teenagers have been declining rapidly. After World War II, birthrates increased in all age groups under 30 years of age. In women aged 20–29 the rate peaked in 1961 and has declined fairly consistently since. Among teenagers the peak came some 10 years later in 1971 and since then the birthrate for the under 20 years age group has declined by 52%, more than in any other age group under age 40 years. The decline in births in teenagers has continued at a slower rate since 1979 and in women aged 25–39 there has been a 'catch-up' effect of births postponed at the younger ages. Between 1971 and 1983 the median age of first nuptial birth increased from 23.7 years to 25.7 years, largely due to the changes in teenage births.

Abortion

It is not enough to consider births alone, we must consider the rate of total pregnancies, based on the actual birthrate and an estimate for the number of abortions.

Estimates, using South Australian abortion data, show that about two thirds of the decline in teenage births has been due to better contraceptive use which has reduced the total number of pregnancies and that one third has been due to an increase in abortion. In addition South Australian abortion data indicate that abortion rates appear to have stabilized since 1980 and may be declining even in teenagers.

Groups who oppose making contraceptive information and services available to teenagers still warn that this will increase teenage promiscuity and pregnancy. Usually these people quote statistics from the USA in the early 70s and ignore Australian statistics and trends which have been markedly different. In 1980, the age specific birthrate in the USA for the age group 15–19 was 53.0 per 1000 population (white 44.7, black 100.00) compared with the Australian rate of 27.6 per 1000 population. Moreover teenage birthrates have declined in the USA . . .

In spite of the decline in teenage births, there is no room for complacency. It is necessary also to look at the components of the decline. The greatest decline has occurred among married teenagers and particularly in those births which result from ex-nuptial conception (births in the first 7 months of marriage) . . .

More Visibility

Teenage pregnancy has become more visible, whereas it was previously hidden behind enforced marriage or clandestine abortion, birth or adoption. One can only wonder at the cruelty imposed on young women who previously faced the trauma of abortion, birth and adoption in secret, often with little social, financial or even family support.

There is now less shame and stigma attached to ex-nuptial birth and single parenthood. Many young women, especially those with family support, cope very well with single parenthood; a surprising number, especially among the older ones, manage to complete their training and even a University course, and take up their careers when their babies have reached school or pre-school age.

The decline in teenage pregnancy and births has flattened out in the past few years and a number of social factors may be responsible. It is likely that there have been two opposing trends—an overall reduction in teenage births, and a sustained or even increasing level among a vulnerable group in the community. Girls who leave school early have less information, fewer job opportunities, lower self esteem, and may be less likely to obtain and make use of contraceptive advice. We know little about the social characteristics of the young women who proceed with an ex-nuptial birth . . .

Disadvantages of Teenage Pregnancy

Statistically, unplanned pregnancy and single parenthood in teenagers carry health, social and financial disadvantages.

The younger the age at first pregnancy the greater the likelihood of further pregnancy and repeat abortion. In 1980, in South Australia, 8.4% of abortions were repeat abortions and 20% of these were in teenage women. Although the serious infections and deaths that followed illegal abortions have now largely disappeared, there still remains a risk of pelvic infection and subsequent infertility that increases with repeated abortions. Early sexual intercourse and changes in sexual partners expose the young woman to the risk of sexually transmitted disease, pelvic infection and possible infertility, and are now recognized as risk factors for cancer of the cervix.

There is still some debate as to whether abortion, especially if repeated, results in cervical incompetence and premature birth in subsequent pregnancies. Pregnant teenagers are more likely to report late for abortion which may necessitate a more complicated and more traumatic procedure . . .

Unplanned pregnancy and single parenthood cause interruption to schooling and job training, reduction in career prospects and interference in what is now regarded as the normal transition to adulthood—workforce experience and independence before marriage and childbearing. Abortion or adoption may be accompanied by psychological stress, guilt and grief particularly, if at a later age, the young woman finds difficulty in conceiving.

Teenage mothers may lack management and parenting skills. Young women on supporting parent benefits are caught in a poverty trap. Only those with good earning capacity can afford to take full-time employment. Others find it a financial disadvantage even to take part-time work. Low income means poor nutrition, limited leisure time activities, disadvantages in housing, and social isolation. Many young women have solved these problems by communal living and mutual support . . .

Access to Contraception

Contraception has only been available to any degree for un-married people since the early 1970s.

There is still some reluctance to prescribe contraception for un-married minors, especially those under age 16. The right of minors to obtain confidential medical advice including contraceptive advice is still under challenge. In the United Kingdom, Mrs. Victoria Gillick last year successfully waged a campaign to prevent doctors prescribing contraceptives for underage girls without informing the parents. The judgement in this case was overturned by the House of Lords in October 1985. There has been no proscription about boys obtaining condoms. In the USA, the so-called 'squeal' rule was narrowly defeated in 1983 and in May 1985 the USA House, Energy and Commerce Committee rejected a proposal to require federally funded clinics to notify parents if their teenage children seek contraception or counselling.

In Australia the legal situation is unclear. In 1976 the Federal Government established the Action Centre in Melbourne to provide confidential advice to adolescents and successive governments have continued this support. At the International Conference on Population, in Mexico, 1984, Australia supported a recommendation that information should be available to teenagers. Although under Medicare, barriers of cost have largely been removed, many teenagers are intimidated from seeking advice from the conventional medical services and authority figures . . .

Conclusion

Major changes have occurred in community attitudes toward pregnancy and single parenthood in teenagers, and teenage pregnancy has become more visible. Continuing trends are a decline in total pregnancies, births and abortions. Adoption or marriage are less likely to be seen as the solution to ex-nuptial conception but pregnancy in teenagers carries health, social and financial risks to both mother and baby. Solutions are not simple and do not depend on the provision of family planning services alone. There needs to also be a broader approach to improving the status, education and career opportunities of women and increased attention to adequate care and support for teenagers, during and after the birth of their children.

8 GLOBAL PERSPECTIVES ON ADOLESCENT PREGNANCY

EARLY PREGNANCY IN BRAZIL AND GUATEMALA

Marilyn Edmunds and John M. Paxman

MULTI-SERVICE CENTER APPROACH —EL CAMINO IN GUATEMALA

Background. Guatemala lies immediately south of Mexico, bordered on its own southern side by Honduras and El Salvador, and to the east by Belize. The Pacific Ocean lies to the southwest. Available census statistics suggest that the total population is between 7 and 7.5 million. Indians who live in the rural areas of the northern and western highlands comprise about half of the population. Spanish is the official language, but these indigenous groups speak as many as twenty different languages.

Severe social and economic problems face the country, and are reflected in high infant mortality rates, high illiteracy rates, low life expectancy rates and significant housing problems. Since the 1950's, Guatemala has been dominated by military rulers, whose reigns have been regularly punctuated by coups d'etat and assassinations of populist leaders. Guerrilla activity has become routine in many areas, further disrupting the possibility of a return to "normalcy." Guatemala City, the capital, is home for the majority of the country's urban dwellers. While residents of the capital city are not as poor as their rural counterparts, unemployment rates are high, coupled with high costs of living.

Marilyn Edmunds and John M. Paxman, "Early Pregnancy and Childbearing," *Pathpapers,* No. 11, September, 1984, pp. 5–10.

The Problem. Like most developing countries, Guatemala has a large population under the age of 20. Recent surveys indicate that 40% of the urban population are 14 and under. Due to the harsh economic circumstances, many young people must drop out of school to seek part-time work in an effort to increase the family income. Adolescents are forced to "grow up" quickly without access to health and social services to help them with problems, such as unplanned pregnancies.

Census data from 1973 documented that 17% of all births were to women 19 years and younger. The same year, the age-specific birth rate for women aged 15–19 was 134 per thousand, and 10.3% of all birth-related maternal deaths were to young women in that age range . . .

In 1978 representatives of APROFAM, the non-profit, national family planning association of Guatemala and local affiliate of International Planned Parenthood Federation, approached The Pathfinder Fund with plans to open a multi-service adolescent center in Guatemala City. Modeled after The Door in New York City, Centro del Adolescente "El Camino" proposed to integrate social services with contraceptive education and services . . .

Client Profile. Fully one-third of the adolescents who visited El Camino during the first year reported serious family difficulties. In addition, one of every four clients faced problems relating to pregnancy, induced abortion and/or a need for contraceptive services. Seven percent received treatment for sexually-transmitted diseases. The two most frequently used services at the center were general psychological counseling and counseling about contraceptive methods. It became evident to the staff that adolescents coming to the center during that year faced a multiplicity of problems requiring a wide range of service interventions.

Program changes. Over time the structure of El Camino's services changed in response to the needs of the adolescents. Arrangements were made with a local university to have advanced psychology students do volunteer placements at the center, which allowed El Camino to offer increased counseling services. A similar agreement later resulted in the addition of dental services. To provide a greater variety of sports and recreational activities, the staff collaborated with the Instituto Nacional de la Juventud, the governmental body which promotes sporting activities for youth. As a result, staff and adolescents were encouraged to participate in national sporting events and could occasionally use official facilities for El Camino events. Finally, a connection was made with the Ministry of Education, which helped to promote El Camino's services within schools and colleges, and also arranged for a limited number of secondary school tuition scholarships for adolescents interested in studying education.

The continuous efforts by El Camino staff to generate local support for the center's activities have met with varying degrees of success. While important contacts have been made, many have also been lost due to political instability and changing leadership which results from periodic shuffling of government positions. Given the extent of economic and political upheaval in Guatemala during the past decade, El Camino has done a remarkable job of acquiring support from national agencies and volunteers.

THE POST-PARTUM HOSPITAL
CLINIC APPROACH—BRAZIL

Background. Brazil, the largest country in Latin America, has a population of over 120 million people, which represents half the total population of the South American continent. Great regional diversity exists throughout Brazil, a result of the wide variety of cultures which have had influence in the country over the centuries. It has been said that Brazil is two countries in one: the underdeveloped North and the industrialized South. The three largest cities, São Paulo, Rio de Janeiro and Belo Horizonte account for nearly half the total population.

The Problem. High population growth rates in the 1960's contributed to Brazil's current youthful population; forty-one percent are under the age of 15. Each year an ever larger cohort of women enter the childbearing years, guaranteeing a steady, if not high, population growth for years to come. Early pregnancies among young women are cause for serious concern, particularly relating to maternal and child health. In 1980 the age-specific birth rate for 15–19 year olds nationwide was 60 per thousand, but in the Northeast part of the country the same rate ranged from 80–100 per thousand. Women in this age group accounted for about 6.8% of births overall, and in the Northeast accounted for 11% of births.

Bahia is one of three states in Northeastern Brazil which still lacks a state supported family planning program. Its age-specific birth rate for 15–19 year olds is 94 per thousand, one of the highest in the nation.

The Clinic. In 1982, the Tsylla Balbino Maternity, a publicly financed hospital that serves predominantly low-income people, opened the first adolescent fertility clinic in Brazil with support from The Pathfinder Fund. Many young women who deliver their babies at the hospital have received no pre-natal care. In addition to deliveries, the hospital treats a large number of patients suffering from complications of induced abortions. About 20% of all patients are aged 19 or younger and many of these women have already had one pregnancy.

Implications. The adolescent clinic is now in its second year of funding from Pathfinder. Indications are that even more patients will be seen in this project year. Data is being collected for an analysis of the clinic's services during the first two years. In addition to gathering data that will profile the average client, information will be sought from clients who have dropped out of the program or discontinued their contraceptive method. Second year plans also include broadening the outreach activities to promote the clinic's service to young women prior to a first, unplanned pregnancy.

The Tsylla Balbino Maternity Adolescent Clinic has come to be regarded as a model for practitioners in other parts of Brazil. Recently, an adolescent clinic was established in the city of Recife, capital of Pernambuco, another state in Northeastern Brazil. The Encruzilhada Maternity Hospital clinic was patterned after the Tsylla Balbino clinic and operates in much the same manner. A group of physicians and nurses from other parts of Brazil who work with adolescents attended a conference on adolescent fertility programs which was sponsored by The Pathfinder Fund and the Tsylla Balbino Maternity Hospital in November 1983. The meeting was held in Salvador, Bahia, giving participants a chance to visit the adolescent clinic and observe its operation. Several of those who attended this conference have since begun planning adolescent programs in their own regions.

WHAT IS EDITORIAL BIAS?

This activity may be used as an individualized study guide for students in libraries and resource centers or as a discussion catalyst in small group and classroom discussions.

The capacity to recognize an author's point of view is an essential reading skill. The skill to read with insight and understanding involves the ability to detect different kinds of opinions or bias. Sex bias, race bias, ethnocentric bias, political bias and religious bias are five basic kinds of opinions expressed in editorials and all literature that attempts to persuade. They are briefly defined below.

5 Kinds of Editorial Opinion or Bias

sex bias— *the expression of dislike for and/or feeling of superiority over the opposite sex or a particular sexual minority*

race bias—the expression of dislike for and/or feeling of superiority over a racial group

ethnocentric bias—the expression of a belief that one's own group, race, religion, culture or nation is superior. Ethnocentric persons judge others by their own standards and values.

political bias—the expression of political opinions and attitudes about domestic or foreign affairs

religious bias—the expression of a religious belief or attitude

Guidelines

1. From the readings in chapter one, locate five sentences that provide examples of editorial opinion or bias.
2. Write down each of the above sentences and determine what kind of bias each sentence represents. Is it sex bias, race bias, ethnocentric bias, political bias or religious bias?
3. Make up one sentence statements that would be an example of each of the following: *sex bias, race bias, ethnocentric bias, political bias* and *religious bias*.
4. See if you can locate five sentences that are factual statements from the readings in chapter one.

CHAPTER 2

PREVENTING TEENAGE PREGNANCY

9   SEX EDUCATION HAS FAILED
    William J. Bennett

10   SEX EDUCATION HAS NOT FAILED
    Karen Sue Smith

11   CONTRACEPTIVES AND THE RISE IN
    PREGNANCIES: POINTS AND
    COUNTERPOINTS
    Howard Hurwitz vs. The Nation

12   SCHOOL BASED CLINICS WILL NOT WORK
    Phyllis Schlafly

13   SCHOOL CLINICS CAN REDUCE PREGNANCY
    RATES
    *Laurie S. Zabin, Marilyn B. Hirsch, Edward
    A. Smith, Rosalie Streett, and Janet B. Hardy*

14   REMOVING ADVERTISING RESTRICTIONS ON
    CONTRACEPTIVES
    The Population Institute

15   CONTRACEPTIVE COMMERCIALS ARE
    INAPPROPRIATE
    Alfred R. Schneider

16   DECEIVING OURSELVES ABOUT SAFE SEX
    Anthony B. Robinson

PREVENTING TEENAGE PREGNANCY

SEX EDUCATION HAS FAILED

William J. Bennett

William J. Bennett is the U.S. Secretary of Education. He delivered this address to the National School Boards Association in Washington, D.C. on January 22, 1987.

Points to Consider

1. Why is the question of character important in a sex education class?
2. What evidence is there that sex education has failed?
3. What is wrong with the way sex education is being taught in the schools?
4. How should teaching be improved?

Excerpted from a speech by William J. Bennett before the National School Boards Association in Washington, DC on January 22, 1987.

The words of morality, of a rational, mature morality, seem to have been banished from sex education.

Today I would like to talk about one place in which attention must be paid to character in an explicit, focused way. That is in the classroom devoted to sex education. It would be undesirable, but a teacher could conduct large portions of a history or English class without explicit reference to questions of character. But to neglect questions of character in a sex-education class would be a great and unforgivable error. Sex education has to do with how boys and girls, how men and women, treat each other and themselves. It has to do with how boys and girls, how men and women, *should* treat each other and themselves. Sex education is therefore about character and the formation of character. A sex-education course in which issues of right and wrong do not occupy center stage is an evasion and an irresponsibility . . .

Sex Education

For several years now I have been looking at the actual form the idea of sex education assumes once it is in the classroom. Having surveyed samples of the literature available to the schools, and having gained a sense of the attitudes that pervade some of the literature, I must say this: I have my doubts. It is clear to me that some programs of sex education are not constructive. In fact, they may be just the opposite. In some places, some people, to be sure, are doing an admirable job. But in all too many places, sex education classes are failing to give the American people what they are entitled to expect for their children, and what their children deserve.

Seventy percent of all high-school seniors had taken sex education courses in 1985, up from 60 percent in 1976. Yet when we look at what is happening in the sexual lives of American students, we can only conclude that it is doubtful that much sex education is doing any good at all. The statistics by which we may measure how our children—how our boys and girls—are treating one another sexually are little short of staggering:

- More than one-half of America's young people have had sexual intercourse by the time they are 17.

- More than one million teen-age girls in the United States become pregnant each year. Of those who give birth, nearly half are not yet 18.
- Teen pregnancy rates are at or near an all-time high. A 25-percent decline in birth rates between 1970 and 1984 is due to a doubling of the abortion rate during that period. More than 400,000 teen-age girls now have abortions each year.
- Unwed teen-age births rose 200 percent between 1960 and 1980.
- Forty percent of today's 14-year-old girls will become pregnant by the time they are 19.

These numbers are, I believe, an irrefutable indictment of sex education's effectiveness in reducing teen-age sexual activity and pregnancies. For these numbers have grown even as sex education has expanded. I do *not* suggest that sex education has *caused* the increase in sexual activity among youth; but clearly it has not prevented it. As Larry Cuban, professor of education at Stanford University, has written: "Decade after decade ... statistics have demonstrated the ineffectiveness of such courses in reducing sexual activity [and] teen-age pregnancy. .... In the arsenal of weapons to combat teen-age pregnancy, school-based programs are but a bent arrow. However, bent arrows do offer the illusion of action." ...

A curriculum guide for one of the largest school systems in the country suggests strategies to "help students learn about their own attitudes and behaviors and find new ways of dealing with problems." For example, students are given the following so-called "problem situation," asked to "improvise dialogue" and "act it out" and then discuss "how everyone felt about the interactions."

Susan and Jim are married. He becomes intoxicated and has sex with his secretary. He contracts herpes, but fails to tell Susan. What will happen in this situation? How would you react if you were Susan and found out? ...

Exploring Options

Now the point I would like to make is that exercises like this deal with very complex, sensitive, personal, serious and often agitated situations—situations that involve human beings at their

62

Sex Ed Aimed at Boys

Although most programs on teenage sexual responsibility are tailored for females, a few are attempting to deal with sexually active teenage boys, according to the Center for Population Options, a Washington clearinghouse on information, research and programs related to teenage sexuality and pregnancy.

Approaches being tried in other cities include: A Chicago program for teenage boys designed to complement the Parents Too Soon program for teenage girls at Rush-Presbyterian-St. Luke's Medical Center. The program provides information on sexually transmitted diseases and homosexuality to younger boys and information on pregnancy, childbirth and contraception to older boys.

Kate Perry, *Minneapolis Star and Tribune,* November 10, 1986

deepest levels. But the guiding pedagogical instruction to teachers in approaching all such "sensitive and personal issues" is this: "Where strong differences of opinion exist on what is right or wrong sexual behavior, objective, informed and dignified discussion of both sides of such questions should be encouraged." And that's it—no more. The curriculum guide is loaded with devices to help students "explore the options," "evaluate the choices involved," "identify alternative actions" and "examine their own values." It provides some facts for students, some definitions, some information, lots of "options"—but that's all.

What's wrong with this kind of teaching? First, it is a very odd kind of teaching—very odd because it does not teach. It does not teach because, while speaking to a very important aspect of human life, it displays a conscious aversion to making moral distinctions. Indeed, it insists on holding them in abeyance. The words of morality, of a rational, mature morality, seem to have been banished from this sort of sex education.

To do what is being done in these classes is tantamount to throwing up our hands and saying to our young people: "We give up. We give up on teaching right and wrong to you. Here, take these facts, take this information, and take your feelings, your options, and try to make the best decisions you can. But you're on your own. We can say no more." It is ironic that, in the part of our children's lives where they may most need adult guidance, and where indeed I believe they most want it, too often the young find instead an abdication of responsible moral authority . . .

Educating About Sex

With these thoughts in mind, I would like to offer a few principles that speak to the task of educating school-children about sex, principles that I believe should inform curricular materials and textbooks, and by which such materials could be evaluated. These principles are, I believe, what most American parents are looking for in sex education.

First, we should recognize that sexual behavior is a matter of character and personality, and that we cannot be value-neutral about it. Neutrality only confuses children, and may lead them to conclusions we wish them to avoid. Specifically, sex education courses should teach children sexual restraint as a standard to uphold and follow.

Second, in teaching restraint, courses should stress that sex is not simply a physical or mechanical act. We should explain to children that sex is tied to the deepest recesses of the personality. We should tell the truth; we should describe reality. We should explain that sex involves complicated feelings and emotions. Some of these are ennobling, and some of them—let us be truthful—can be cheapening of one's own finer impulses and a cheapening to others.

Third, sex education courses should speak up for the institution of the family. To the extent possible, when they speak of sexual activity, courses should speak of it in the context of the institution of marriage. We should speak of the fidelity, commitment and maturity of successful marriages as something for which our students should strive.

To the girls, teachers need to talk about the readiness for motherhood. And they must do more. They must not be afraid to use words like "modesty" and "chastity." Teachers and curriculum planners must be sure that sex-education courses do not undermine the values and beliefs that still lead most girls to see

64

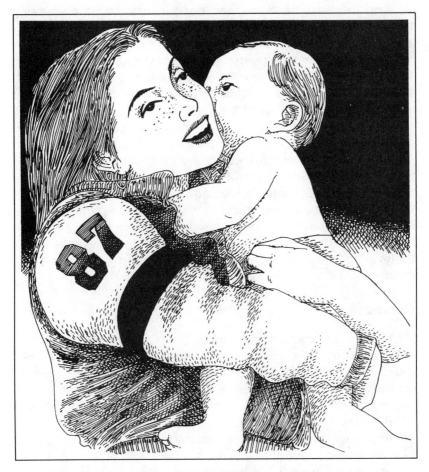

Illustration by Craig MacIntosh. Reprinted by permission of *Star Tribune, Newspaper of the Twin Cities*.

sexual modesty as a good thing. For it is a good thing, and a good word. Let us from time to time praise modesty. And teachers must not be afraid to teach lessons other girls have learned from bitter experience. They should quote Lani Thompson, from T. C. Williams High School in Alexandria, Va., who says of some of her friends: "I get upset when I see friends losing their virginity to some guy they've just met. Later, after the guy's dumped them, they come to me and say, 'I wish I hadn't done it.' "

And the boys need to hear these things too. In discussing these matters, teachers should not forget to talk to the boys. They should tell the boys what it is to be a father, what it is to be ready to be a father, what the responsibilities of being a father are. And they should tell them how the readiness and responsibility of being a father should precede or at least accompany the acts which might make them fathers.

Fourth, sex-education courses should welcome parents and other adults as allies. They should welcome parents into sex-education classrooms as observers. If they do not, I would be suspicious. They should inform parents of the content of these courses, and they should encourage parents and children to talk to each other about sex. Studies show that when parents are the main source of sex education, children are less likely to engage in sex. This should come as no surprise when one remembers that the home is the crucible of character and that parents are children's first and foremost teachers.

Conclusion

Many parents admit that they do not do enough to teach their children about sex. But parents, more than anyone else, still make the difference. Sex-education courses can help remind those parents of their responsibilities. And these courses should encourage the individual counsel of priests, ministers, rabbis and other adults who know a child well and who will take the time and offer the advice needed for that particular child. For it is the quality of the care and time that individuals take with other individuals that means the most in the formation of character.

Finally, schools, parents and communities should pay attention to who is teaching their children about sex. They should remember that teachers are role models for young people. And so it is crucial that sex-education teachers offer examples of good character by the way they act, and by the ideals and convictions they must be willing to articulate to students. As Oxford University's Mary Warnock has written: "You cannot teach morality without being committed to morality yourself; and you cannot be committed to morality yourself without holding that some things are right and others wrong."

These, then, are some of the principles I would like to see standing behind our schools' sex-education courses. The truth, of course, is that what I think in this matter isn't as important as what you think. I don't have any schools. You've got the schools, and part of your job is to help inform the philosophies that guide them. Above all else, then, I would urge you, as you think about those philosophies, to make sure your schools are teaching our children the truth. Sometimes the simplest way to recognize the truth is to consult common sense. Let me urge you to follow your common sense. Don't be intimidated by the sexologists, by the so-called sex-ed experts, by the sex technicians. Character education is mostly a matter of common sense. If sex-education courses are prepared to deal with the truth, with reality in all its complexity, with the hard truths of the human condition, then they should be welcome in our schools. But if sex-education courses are not prepared to tell the truth, if instead they want to simplify or distort or omit certain aspects of these realities in this very important realm of human life, then we should let them go out of business. If sex-education courses do not help in the effort to provide an education in character, then let them be gone from the presence of our children.

PREVENTING TEENAGE PREGNANCY

SEX EDUCATION HAS NOT FAILED

Karen Sue Smith

Karen Sue Smith is an assistant editor of Commonweal *magazine.*

Points to Consider

1. Why did foes of sex education lose an eloquent spokesman?
2. What are the grim facts about teen sexual activity in the U.S.?
3. What objections do critics raise about the nature of sex education in the schools?
4. What kind of consensus should be reached between the critics and opponents of sex education?

Karen Sue Smith, "Sex Education: A Matter of Body and Soul," *Commonweal,* April 10, 1987, pp. 206–10.

Koop suggested not only that sex education is essential, but that, in light of the AIDS crisis, explicit information about heterosexual and homosexual behavior should be included in school curricula.

Last October, foes of sex education lost an eloquent spokesman. Surgeon General C. Everett Koop fanned an already inflamed national controversy about sex education in public schools. Koop suggested not only that sex education is essential, but that, in light of the AIDS crisis, explicit information about heterosexual and homosexual behavior should be included in school curricula.

What should be included in the curriculum? Who should decide? What is the role of parents, health care professionals, and religious leaders? How will these decisions be made, given our pluralistic society? These are some of the questions that have ignited the sex education debate around the nation. And while it may not be a typical example, New York City—with its ethnic and religious diversity, reputation for the cultural avant garde, and sheer size—makes an instructive case study.

New York Curriculum

The same month Koop made his speech, all seven members of the New York City Board of Education voted to require every public school to implement a sex education program, using as a base the revised curriculum, "Family Living Including Sex Education." The Board's mandate gave foes of the city curriculum a rallying cry. Opponents mounted a campaign to have the curriculum withdrawn and still further revised even though:

● the curriculum, in earlier editions, has been in place since 1967;

● the revised third edition has been reviewed by an advisory committee composed of community leaders including clergy;

● the curriculum has been piloted in four elementary districts (two heavily Roman Catholic) and several high schools over a four-year period without major, irreconcilable objections;

● the program has been voluntarily implemented by twenty-one out of thirty-two city elementary districts and all high schools;

69

- the curriculum may be adapted by local districts, modifications subject to the approval of the chancellor;
- the directives insist that an advisory committee for each school and district review the program annually;
- any parent may request, by signing a waiver, that his or her child be withdrawn from the course.

Naturally, the city looks upon the activities of its critics as an effort to reopen a closed case. This September, the curriculum is scheduled to be in place.

The most organized and vocal opponents of the plan include the Roman Catholic Archdiocese of New York, the Diocese of Brooklyn, and an ad hoc group, the Coalition of Concerned Clergy, who wrote an open letter to the Board last December. The letter was signed by diocesan officials plus several vicars, one rabbi, a few Orthodox priests, and a score of evangelical clergy. Curiously, not one mainline Protestant was among the signatories, unless one were to stretch the term to include Richard Neuhaus, who was a signer. Nor was the coalition, East Brooklyn Churches, listed, a well organized group of activists known for bending the ear of City Hall until hundreds of housing units had been erected in their community.

Publicly, the archdiocese makes clear that it is not opposed to sex education per se. (As early as 1965 the Vatican document, "Declaration on Christian Education," admonished teachers that as children "grow older they should receive positive and prudent education in matters relating to sex.") Rather, it is this particular curriculum which dioceses reject. The overarching objection is one applicable to programs around the country (and is not limited to sex education): the value-free pretensions of the curriculum.

In an op ed piece for *Newsday* (January 8, 1987) Msgr. John G. Woolsey wrote: "The curriculum is devoid of moral values and premises. It conveys information about sexuality in a mechanical fashion and a purely secular vocabulary." Woolsey cites "sexual abstinence, chastity, modesty, and marital fidelity" as terms noticeably absent from the city's course.

A lack of values, critics say, lies at the heart of the curriculum's hesitancy to say when sexual activity is appropriate and when it is not; which family pattern should be presented as the ideal; whether or not homosexuality is just one mode of sexual expression among others; which contraceptive methods are preferable, and so on . . . .

Reality and Ideals

Reality and ideals. It is the relation between them that forms the core of the dispute over values in education generally, and sex education in particular.

On the one hand, it is the staggering realities of a generation of social upheaval and rapid change—affecting sexual activity (with all its ramifications), marriage, family structures, and social tolerances—which public school teachers face daily. Regardless of what people say their values are, the facts are grim.

An article by Gary L. Bauer in the *Washington Post* (January 5, 1987) listed these statistics:

● 14 percent of children who began school in September, 1986 have unmarried parents;

● 40 percent will live in a broken home before they reach their eighteenth birthday;

● between one-quarter and one-third are latchkey children.

● Births out of wedlock, as a percentage of all births, increased more than 450 percent in just thirty years.

● Child and spouse abuse has climbed to its highest level since accurate polling began measuring it.

Add to this a divorce rate at around 50 percent; a poverty rate among single mothers and their children—the economic factor inextricably intertwined with teen pregnancy—that is growing faster than that of any other group. Finally, there is the high rate among teens of sexually transmitted diseases, the life and death specter of AIDS, and a rising rate of teen suicide.

These realities raise a host of questions for educators: If low self-esteem is a major contributor to premature sexual activity, pregnancy, and anti-social behavior among youth, can the school foster a healthy self-image among its students by holding up expectations for family life that half its students' families fail to exemplify? Will emphasizing the stable, two-parent model of family (an emphasis critics want) help students cope with parental divorce and other painful family changes they are facing? The argument is that such an ideal serves to undervalue the accomplishments of a happy "reconstituted" family—husband, wife, and children from a previous marriage—or the sacrifices of the mother who has successfully raised her family alone . . .

Two Values

The two values that critics of the curriculum seem to mention most consistently are: that the traditional two-parent, stable family structure be presented as the achievable ideal, not one option among others, and that sexual activity outside of marriage be taught clearly as wrong. Indeed, critics have charged that the curriculum is not merely morally vacuous, but that sexual activity by children and teens is treated as "acceptable" behavior; it may even be encouraged by the program. A position paper drawn up by the Office of Catholic Education, Diocese of Brooklyn, describes what it calls "the philosophical underpinning of the curriculum": Boys and girls, beginning around the fifth grade become sexually active and continue to be so with a variety of partners both homosexual and heterosexual throughout the rest of their lives. This behavior is acceptable as long as no one becomes pregnant or contracts a sexually transmitted disease. Girls should know that should they become pregnant, abortion is an alternative which they may choose without the knowledge or consent of their parents.

A reading of the pilot edition of the curriculum shows that critics do have a point: the curriculum manages, for the most part, to avoid making moral pronouncements—saying what is right or wrong—even on issues for which it reserves its strongest language. A convincing case can be made, and ought to be made, that the language used is too weak in its attempts to present the disadvantages of sexual activity by children and

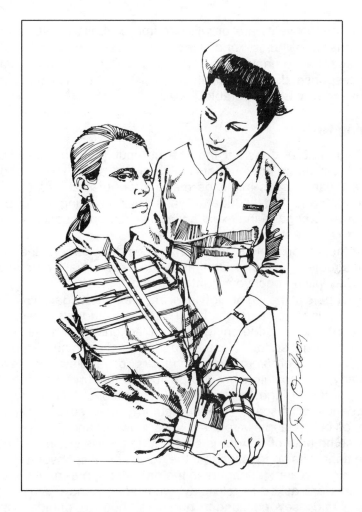

teens—especially given the amount of time and space allotted to contraception, pregnancy, and sexually transmitted diseases. Several of the concrete recommendations along these lines by the diocese would significantly improve the curriculum; most notably, an insertion at strategic places in the text of the question: Why is it important not to engage in sexual intercourse as a young teen?

Having said this, it is only fair to add that the diocesan statement above is an overstatement, a serious misrepresentation of the spirit and letter of the curriculum. The schools simply have to recognize the fact that some children (hundreds of thousands of them each year) are or will become sexually active in their preteens and teens, and they must teach students about contraception, prenatal care, and disease. But such a recognition and response does not, in itself, constitute a philosophy that sexual activity is "acceptable."

Saying No

Furthermore, consider that the curriculum includes lessons called "saying no" for students in fifth grade through high school. While these lessons might be made stronger and clearer, they do encourage "abstinence" of a sort—not giving in to peer pressure to engage in sexual activity—even on occasions when they do not mention the term directly.

In the lesson for fifth and sixth grades, for example, teachers are instructed to emphasize that "when people really care about you, they will respect your right to say no."

Teachers at the junior high level are cautioned against making "censorious statements which will decrease students' feelings of self-worth," and condemning parental actions "which may differ from traditional codes." Yet the teacher is asked to help students examine the *problems and dangers* of adolescent sexual intimacy, and to "highlight the positive values of love, commitment, and marriage." For reasons of emotional immaturity, not pregnancy or disease, the curriculum says, sexual intimacy among young people is referred to as "unwise" and "dangerous." (The same note of danger is sounded in the New York bishops' statement in its suggestion that the government sponsor a media campaign "to alert teenagers to the dangers of pre-marital sex.") Students are asked to role play, write about, and discuss how they would "say no" under pressure; how to decide which behavior is best when peer values conflict with parental values; and to think ahead about how decisions they make now will affect the future . . .

Reaching Consensus

Currently, diocesan campaigns are being waged to assure that parents and clergy are informed of the issues and to encourage them and other parishioners to volunteer to serve on school district and local school advisory committees. Packets of materials are being distributed to pastors and administrators.

They contain detailed lists of problem areas within the curriculum; a position paper applying church teaching to the proposed curriculum; a copy of the health clinic parental consent form; and an annotated dissection of typical Board arguments used on behalf of the sex ed program in meetings with parents.

Whether the Board will be willing to make major changes at this point in time remains to be seen, but the basic debate on values may continue with each yearly review.

While it looks like a battle, the process itself could be valuable. If parents respond positively, and if appeals to them are neither alarmist nor distorted, discussion could remind parents that the sexual education of their children is primarily their own responsibility. If parents are ill-equipped for the job, the church and school can help them. Furthermore, the expectation within the curriculum—that students already arrive at school with values planted and cultivated by home, church, and synagogue—should challenge Catholic parents, clergy, and educators to make sure this assumption is valid.

Consensus will require not only honesty and dialogue, but a willingness to give and take. Maybe it will mean including more lessons and stronger language about postponing sex for children and teens. This is a value that could be agreed upon by a diverse constituency for a variety of psychological, physiological, social, and moral reasons which involve no religious imposition of any kind. But to reject a public school curriculum until it teaches that sex should be postponed until marriage—that is, to expect it to teach the value of life-long chastity and sexual intercourse only within marriage (as the church teaches but the society at large does not espouse or practice)—is to prevent a consensus on the curriculum as a whole. The costs of such an impasse should be carefully weighed. If consensus can be reached on strongly discouraging students' sexual activity, it would be worth a tradeoff of some lesser objection Catholic critics and others might have.

Those who criticize the curriculum for its "morality by consensus" approach to issues are correct about one thing: morality itself is not determined by consensus. But the values which are to be included in a public school curriculum certainly are.

PREVENTING TEENAGE PREGNANCY

CONTRACEPTIVES AND THE RISE IN PREGNANCIES: POINTS AND COUNTERPOINTS

Howard Hurwitz vs. *The Nation* Magazine

The following counterpoints were taken from Human Events, *a conservative journal of social and political thought and* The Nation, *a liberal publication.*

Points to Consider

1. How many New York City schools dispense contraceptives?
2. What is the likelihood that condom distribution will stem the rising tide of teen pregnancies?
3. What has happened to teen pregnancy rates in schools with school-based clinics?
4. What nations have the lowest rate of pregnancy?
5. What are the solutions to teen pregnancy?

Howard Hurwitz, "Contraceptives for New York City Students," *Human Events,* November 29, 1986, p. 17 and "Papa Don't Preach," *The Nation* magazine, The Nation Company, Inc., © October 25, 1986.

THE POINT—by Howard Hurwitz

Basic education is being expanded to include distribution of condoms to high school students. At one New York City high school, the condoms are displayed on the shelves of the health clinic in the school. Ask and you shall receive is the counsel of the principal. Along with other defenders of school distribution of contraceptive devices, he sees it as the means of preventing teenage pregnancies.

Data

Data collected by the Washington-based, private Center for Population Options show 61 such school clinics. Ten of them, including two in New York City, dispense contraceptives, and 39 more, including one in New Haven and seven in New York City, have physicians who can write prescriptions for birth control pills or devices.

The revelation that New York City high schools have been in the condom business (non-profit) for over a year took the bachelor president of the Board of Education by surprise. He learned about it accidentally, when he read a report on sex education that was given to him by the schools chancellor.

Both board president and chancellor have been scurrying around for safe positions. Board President Robert Wagner Jr., son of a former mayor, has decided for the moment that the condoms should be given to students who are 18. Chancellor Nathan Quinones believes that the condoms should be distributed only to those students whose parents sign a consent form.

Condom Distribution

Both seem unaware that condom distribution, and contraception education in the curriculum, require homework by the students. Homework is not always done carefully by students, and there is little reason to believe that greater care will be taken by students in the contraceptive course.

Now that the cover has been ripped off the undercover Board of Education involvement in condom distribution, the notoriety will not be confined to DuSable High School in Chicago or the much-touted Baltimore anti-pregnancy campaign. DuSable has been picketed by critics, but the condom kids go about their business.

In New York, the black principal of the almost all-black Boys-Girls High School has come out against condom clinics. He sees the schools selected for the service as predominantly minority in enrollment. If his vision improves, he may see that 80 per cent of the nearly one million children in New York City's 1,000 public schools are minority members. If there should be a real burst of light, he may see that teenage pregnancy is not the exclusive right of minorities.

Sexual Practice

Bungled pre-marital teenage sexual practice cuts across racial and ethnic and economic lines. Some 3,000 girls are impregnated daily, according to Secretary of Health and Human Services Otis R. Bowen.

You might think from the rush to open new condom outlets in the public schools that the device is as strange to today's youth as the dodo bird to ornithologists. The condom has been around for over a half-century. The teenager who does not know of its existence requires a different kind of medical counseling. The recommendation by counselors that girls carry them in their purses is of a piece with gun control.

The likelihood that condom distribution in high schools will stem the rising tide of pregnancies is as remote as ordering of the tides without the gravitational attraction by sun and moon. Far more likely is that school approval of condoms, implicit in their distribution, will confirm for students the widely held belief that doing what comes naturally need not be curbed by respect for traditional family living.

Responsibility

Family responsibility is the last thought of youths, who know they are doing wrong, but know also that society either smirks at their precocity, or rushes succor in the form of welfare aid, infant-care centers for teenage mothers in school, and don't-do-it-a-third-time counseling by "trained" teachers.

Is there anyone in the house for chastity? Is there anyone around who believes that premarital sex for school kids is immoral and can be dangerous to their health? Is there anyone left who believes that family living can be taught in class without prescriptions for condoms and pills?

You are out there, all right, but largely out of it. Get organized, before our schools are named after Sodom and Gomorrah.

THE COUNTERPOINT—by The Nation

Last week the New York City Board of Education voted to cut back a pilot program through which health clinics in nine high schools had prescribed, and one had distributed, contraceptives to students. Several board members joined the Roman Catholic Archdiocese in arguing that giving advice on birth control to teen-agers encourages promiscuity. Board president Robert F. Wagner Jr. agrees to limit the provision of contraceptives on school grounds to students 18 and over. This compromise will supposedly protect younger students' morality; it actually means they will be less likely to practice birth control.

At the same time, a clinic based in a Chicago high school has been sued by a group of thirteen black clergymen and a handful of students and parents. They make the demagogic charge that the distribution of contraceptives at the all-black DuSable High School is "a calculated, pernicious effort to destroy the very fabric of family life among black parents and their children." Another party to the suit is the Pro-Life/Pro-Family Coalition, a group that apparently opposes birth control as well as abortion. Their victory would endanger all school-based clinics.

According to the Center for Population Options, the number of school-based clinics offering family planning and other health care has increased from twelve in 1980 to sixty-one today, with another hundred expected to open soon. At least ten dispense contraceptives directly, and about forty more are staffed by physicians who can write prescriptions for birth control pills or devices. Schools with these clinics have reported a marked decline in the rate of student pregnancy.

The problem of teen-age pregnancy in America is acute. In New York City alone, 14,300 women 17 and younger became pregnant in 1985, including 1,240 pregnancies to girls under 15. In 1985, more than 1 million women between the ages of 15 and 19 got pregnant, and over half of them carried their babies to term. Teen-age mothers are far more likely than their childless peers to drop out of school and to end up living in poverty. Of women under 30 who receive Aid to Families with Dependent Children, about 60 percent were teen-agers when they had their first child. Meanwhile, Madonna's hymn to adolescent motherhood tops the charts.

For a brief period last year, children having children made the front pages, but the hype had little impact on Federal priorities. No wonder, since the best way to combat teen-age pregnancy runs counter to the conservative agenda. According to an international study of family planning policies by the Alan Guttmacher Institute, the lowest rates of teen-age pregnancy were in countries that made contraceptives accessible to young people at low cost or for free, without parental notification, and offered sex education.

A detailed survey conducted last year by the House Select Committee on Children, Youth and Families reported that in most states "existing prevention and assistance services are inadequate." Achieving adequacy requires more money than states alone can easily raise. It also requires officials willing to stand up to the right-wingers who would sacrifice the prospects of millions of young women to their fantasies about what America should be.

PREVENTING TEENAGE PREGNANCY

SCHOOL-BASED CLINICS WILL NOT WORK

Phyllis Schlafly

Phyllis Schlafly is the author and publisher of The Phyllis Schlafly Report, *and a leading conservative spokesperson for conservative ideas and causes.*

Points to Consider

1. What is the purpose of school-based sex clinics?
2. What are the health service professionals teaching?
3. How should sex education courses be taught?
4. Why is the "Sex Respect Curriculum" a good alternative to the present sex education curriculums?
5. How are the costs and liabilities described?

Phyllis Schlafly, "School-Based Sex Clinics vs. Sex Respect," *The Phyllis Schlafly Report,* June, 1986, pp. 1–4.

Is it realistic to believe that teenagers can be taught to abstain from premarital sex? Of course it is; that was the pattern for most teenagers until the last 20 years when "sex education" invaded public schools and pornography invaded primetime television.

A radical concept has been propelled by the argument that teenagers are promiscuous anyway (the euphemism is "sexually active"), and therefore the schools should teach them how to avoid having babies. These school-based sex clinics and courses teach a strange new definition of the word responsible: "responsible sexuality" means enjoying promiscuity without guilt and without having a baby.

The promoters of sex clinics for schoolchildren are imposing on a captive audience their peculiar concepts, namely, that promiscuity is good but pregnancy is bad. They are saying, step right up, teenager, and get your contraceptives here; have fun with your sex partner; the only thing that's wrong is having a baby.

About 30 such sex clinics have been quietly (even surreptitiously) introduced into public high schools in recent years. By October 1985, the promoters of this new industry felt confident enough to stage a national conference in Chicago to train hundreds of health service professionals who want to co-opt the schools as rent-free offices for their expanding bureaucracy.

The forces advocating sex clinics have wide access to foundation money and favorable media. CBS's *60 Minutes* gave Planned Parenthood a full segment in April 1986 to propagandize for sex clinics, omitting the usual hostile interruptions. Sex clinics were endorsed on NBC's *Today* Show on May 15, with Bryant Gumbel falsely saying, "there is no opposition."

The plan to install school-based sex clinics was criticized by Education Secretary William J. Bennett on April 11 as an "abdication of moral authority." He said that these clinics "legitimate" sexual activity while encouraging teenagers to have "sexual intimacy on their minds."

Planned Parenthood and the health service professionals, who have a vested interest in providing costly taxpayer-financed "services" to an ever-expanding constituency of "clients," have a typical knee-jerk response. David Andrews, executive vice president of the Planned Parenthood Federation, answers that we face the alternatives of "ignorance" or "pregnancies."

A New Sex Kit

Out of the garbage heap of how-to sex kits, pornography, and contraceptives now being thrust upon school chidren around the country, something beautiful has grown. It's called the "Sex Respect" course, and it's based on an old but radical idea: Teach kids the value of chastity, and means to achieve it, rather than inculcating safe physical techniques of promiscuity.

This fresh breeze is the work of Colleen Kelly Mast, a former teacher and an expert in health education. Mast's program, developed under a grant from the Department of Health and Human Services, is already approved for use in the classroom in most states, and indeed, has been tested extensively around the country.

Gregory A. Fossedal, *Human Events*, June 27, 1987

Those are NOT the alternatives. The correct alternative is for the schools to teach teenagers NOT to engage in premarital sex. When we dare to say that, the liberals and sex-clinic promoters make predictable replies.

First, they say, "That's impossible because it won't work." To which we should answer, "You cannot know that because it hasn't been tried." Ever since sex education was introduced into public schools about 30 years ago, these courses have taught schoolchildren how to do it but have censored out all judgmental warnings against premarital sex.

Second, they say, "That's impossible because teenagers are sexually active anyway." To which we should answer, "A minority of teenagers are, but the majority are not. If the school legitimizes the immoral behavior of the minority, the school will be validating promiscuity by the majority."

Third, they say, "You can't impose your moral values on schoolchildren by telling them that premarital sex is wrong because that would breach the wall of separation of church and state." To which, we should answer, "Nonsense. There isn't any constitutional difference between teaching teenagers that it's wrong to have a baby and teaching them that it's wrong to engage in premarital sex. There isn't any constitutional difference between teaching teenagers that it's wrong to drive a car without a driver's license and teaching them that it's wrong to engage in sex without a marriage license."

Sex Education?

There are many true and powerful reasons to justify teaching abstinence to teenagers without ever mentioning religion or right-or-wrong morality. The schools can teach students that promiscuity is bad, risky, unhealthy, and stupid (especially for girls) because its consequences can be incurable VD, emotional trauma, and a forfeiture of opportunities for a lifetime marriage to a faithful spouse and for career and economic advancement.

This nation has accepted all sorts of government restraints on our personal behavior that are not nearly so dangerous as teenage promiscuity. The seat-belt law and the 55-mile speed limit law are two examples. Teenage promiscuity is more dangerous to more people, and more costly for all of us, than violations of either of those laws.

Yet the public schools are aiding and abetting promiscuity in most of their so-called "sex education" courses. Here is a typical example. The following quotations are from the textbook used since 1978 in the Seattle, Washington, public high schools in a mandatory "Health" course: "Premarital sexual intercourse is acceptable for both men and women if they are involved in a stable loving relationship. It has been suggested by some marriage counseling authorities that all couples should live together before they are married."

"Often promiscuity is labeled as 'bad' by persons who do not accept this type of behavior. As with other patterns of sexual behavior, one should not pin a 'good' or 'bad' label on a practice."

"Morality is individual; it is what YOU think it is. Your conception of what is right or wrong (morality) is an individual decision."

Reading further in this textbook called *You and Your Health* by William Fassbender, we find that it includes pornographic pictures and also teaches:

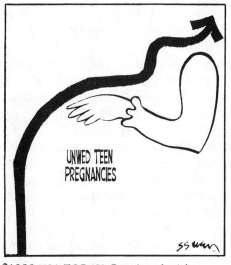

©1985 USA TODAY. Reprinted with permission.

- that homosexuality is a normal lifestyle—and that "gay rights" legislation should be enacted to stop "discrimination" against homosexuals and lesbians;
- that prostitution should be legalized;
- that it is NOT deviant for teenagers to watch others performing sex acts through binoculars, windows, or holes in walls;
- that "alternatives to traditional marriage" include "open marriage where outside sexual relationships can exist and will not harm the marriage," *and* "group marriage" where three or more people live together and "have sexual relations with each other." The textbook asks the student: "Do you feel that you might be interested in becoming a part of such a group? " . . .

Sex Respect

Now there is a new course for junior high schoolers that teaches teenagers how and why to say "no" to sex before marriage. This *Sex Respect* curriculum is currently being piloted in Chicago and St. Louis schools.

With creative lesson plans, cartoons, and jargon that appeal to teenagers, *Sex Respect* gives teenagers the confidence and knowledge to practice sexual abstinence. From a basic health

85

(physical and emotional) perspective, teenagers learn why chastity is the positive and healthy alternative to the "popular contraceptive mentality."

The curriculum includes ten lesson plans and is available in three parts from Project Sex Respect, P.O. Box 39, Golf, Illinois 60029. The price is $10.95 for the teacher's manual, $6.95 for the student workbook, $7.95 for the parent's guide, or $23 for the set of three books, plus $3.50 for postage and handling.

Is it realistic to believe that teenagers can be taught to abstain from premarital sex? Of course it is; that was the pattern for most teenagers until the last 20 years when "sex education" invaded public schools and pornography invaded primetime television. Even the American Association of Sex Educators, Counselors and Therapists heard a speaker at its 1986 convention in Los Angeles say that, if AIDS spreads from homosexuals to heterosexuals, this could "send the nation's sexual mores back to the 1950s, when young people went steady, got engaged and later maintained a monogamous marriage."

Pill Goes To School

"Pill Goes To School" was the way the Chicago Sun-Times broke the news to Chicago area residents that DuSable Public High School has been aiding and abetting promiscuity of schoolchildren by handing out free contraceptives. The news shocked citizens, parents, and teachers, and opposition to the sex clinic has been rising ever since.

The nationwide plan to put free contraceptives in all public schools as soon as financing can be arranged was unveiled at a national conference called "School-Based Health Clinics" in Chicago in October 1985. The several hundred conferees were taken to inspect the DuSable operation as a "model." The plan is to launch the sex clinics with money from big foundations, and then load the costs onto the backs of the taxpayers; the conferees were told that funds could come from 57 federal agencies. The plan is to use the poor (usually in ghetto neighborhoods) as guinea pigs for this social experiment and then impose it on all public schools.

As more and more information surfaces about the sex clinic controversy in Chicago, it has become apparent that there is a vast array of well-known social service organizations, using charitable contributions and foundation money, which has been "networking" in order to "sensitize" communities to the asserted "need" for school-based clinics. Even the American Red Cross, known to the public for its good works in blood banks and disaster relief, is deep into the promotion of school-based sex programs. The goal is to expand the social service bureaucracy and turn the schools into sites to dispense socialized medicine from the cradle to the grave . . .

Costs and Liabilities

The cost of installing and staffing school-based sex clinics is only one of its burdens. An even bigger cost factor may be the financial liability which is incurred by the schools and their school boards. Schools that dispense contraceptives to teenagers may be held financially liable for the venereal disease and other traumas of promiscuity in the same way that the tavern owner can be held liable for auto accidents of persons to whom he serves liquor.

Venereal diseases are at an epidemic level in the United States as a consequence of the sexual revolution, the Playboy mentality, and the prevalence of pornography in entertainment media. Since "sex education" courses started in schools about 30 years ago, they have taught directly or indirectly the lie that antibiotics can cure all venereal diseases.

Today, 20 million Americans have incurable venereal herpes, 4.6 million have chlamydia (which causes infertility among women), and 20,000 have the incurable fatal AIDS. Teenagers who are given contraceptives so they can be "safe" from pregnancy are simply NOT safe from VD, and the school could be held liable for the horrendous costs of these diseases . . .

Even before sex clinics and AIDS came along, public schools faced dramatic increases in the costs of their liability insurance. Many school districts and local government bodies have had their liability insurance canceled or their premiums increased tenfold as a result of a flood of lawsuits and large personal injury settlements. This rise in insurance costs means either curtailing services which some people regard as essential or whopping tax increases to pay the costs.

The sex clinic at DuSable High School sent home a parental consent notice which commits the School-Based Clinic "to provide comprehensive health services" including "Treatment of sexually transmitted diseases." The question Chicago parents are asking is, does existing school health insurance cover this sex clinic and the treatment of venereal diseases (including AIDS) and, if so, how much will school insurance costs skyrocket?

Sample Letter to Schools

It's time for parents and taxpayers to call a halt to the promotion of promiscuity by the public schools. Here is a sample letter that anyone can send to local public schools. All public schools operate with taxpayers' money, and all materials should be open and available to public scrutiny.

Dear Principal:

The news media have reported that there is a nationwide plan to put sex clinics in public schools to dispense contraceptives. I would appreciate a reply to the following questions.

1. Do you have any plan to start a clinic in your school that would dispense contraceptives or prescriptions for contraceptives?

2. If so, who bears the financial liability for medical malpractice, complications from contraceptives and from abortions, and Sexually Transmitted Diseases?

3. Please send me a copy of the Parental Consent Form and any psychological questionnaires to be used by this clinic.

4. Regardless of your answers to the above, please tell me when I may come and see the textbooks and other materials (including films) used by your school that pertain to sexual activity, contraceptives, abortion, and homosexuality.

Thank you for your cooperation.

Sincerely,

PREVENTING TEENAGE PREGNANCY

SCHOOL CLINICS CAN REDUCE PREGNANCY RATES

Laurie S. Zabin, Marilyn B. Hirsch, Edward A. Smith, Rosalie Streett and Janet B. Hardy

Laurie S. Zabin is director of the Social Science Fertility Research Unit in the Department of Gynecology and Obstetrics at the Johns Hopkins University School of Medicine, and Marilyn B. Hirsch and Edward A. Smith are assistant professors in the same department. Rosalie Streett is director of the Community Adolescent Health Center, and Janet B. Hardy is professor emeritus in the Department of Pediatrics, The Johns Hopkins University School of Medicine.

Points to Consider

1. What was the nature of the school based pregnancy prevention program?
2. How did the program affect pregnancy rates?
3. What changes were noted in the area of contraceptive knowledge?
4. What behavior changes were observed?
5. Was the program more successful with older or younger students?

Reproduced with permission from *Family Planning Perspectives*, Vol. 18, Number 3, May/June 1986.

It was the accessibility of the staff and of the clinic, rather than any "new" information about contraception, that encouraged the students to obtain services.

In this article, we report on a school-based program for the primary prevention of pregnancy among inner-city adolescents that was designed and administered by the staff of The Johns Hopkins School of Medicine's Department of Pediatrics and Department of Gynecology and Obstetrics. The project was carried out with the cooperation of the administrators of four schools in the Baltimore school system—two junior high schools and two senior high schools. The program provided the students attending one of the junior high schools and one of the senior high schools with sexuality and contraceptive education, individual and group counseling, and medical and contraceptive services over a period of almost three school years. Students in the remaining two schools received no such services, but provided baseline and end-of-project data, and serve as the control sample . . .

Pregnancy Rates

What effect, if any, do clinic attendance and contraceptive practice have on pregnancy rates? . . .

Pregnancy data were subjected to many types of analysis, including examinations of pregnancies in consecutive 12-month periods and comparison of differentials by outcome of pregnancy. All confirmed the conclusion that the program led to decreases in the pregnancy rates of these 9th–12th-grade students.

Because the numbers of sexually active students in the seventh and eighth grades were small, and because we have much more limited information on their pregnancies, it is difficult to evaluate changes among these students. There appear, however, to be small reductions in pregnancy rates among girls 15 years old and younger.

Concurrently, however, larger increases in pregnancy rates appear to have taken place in the nonprogram schools. We believe, therefore, that the program assisted these younger

Teens Support Sex Education

More than 100 teenagers, many of whom are parents, met at the Washington Convention Center yesterday to discuss sex and teenage pregnancy . . . The students overwhelmingly supported school-based health clinics and suggested better sex education be included in their school curriculums, including more about the meaning of love and what makes relationships work.

Patrice Gaines-Carter, *Washington Post,* April 4, 1986

teenagers in avoiding the kinds of increases observed citywide, and even led to some decrease in their pregnancies.

Two Baltimore Schools

The brief, though intensive, pregnancy prevention program introduced in two Baltimore schools has demonstrated significant changes in several areas of adolescent knowledge and behavior —changes that have major implications for the formulation of public policy and for program design. The results reported in this article are based on the school populations as a whole, and do not compare the individuals who used the program services with those who did not. It is highly noteworthy, therefore, that the differentials are nonetheless statistically significant, and reflect a broad impact on the school community.

Over the course of the two and a half years that the program existed, changes in sexual and contraceptive knowledge occurred. These are both areas in which it has already been demonstrated that educational programs can make a difference. The rapid effect on clinic use exerted by an intervention program designed to supplement the basic sex education program already in place suggests that it was the accessibility of the staff and of the clinic, rather than any "new" information about contraception, that encouraged the students to obtain services.

Our study has shown attitudes to be somewhat more resistant to change than practice, but in this area there was less room for change to occur. As we reported earlier, support for adolescent childbearing or for casual sex was already very low in this school population before the program began. This seemed to suggest that more overall improvement was to be gained by helping students holding positive attitudes toward pregnancy prevention translate those attitudes into action than by attempting to change the attitudes of the few who do not share that view. With majority opinion already supportive of contraception and delayed child-bearing, that is apparently what the program accomplished.

Early Sexual Activity

While the changes in the age at first intercourse are not large, they are substantial enough—in the direction of delay—to refute charges that access to such services as those provided by the program encourages early sexual activity. The program's ability to effect any further changes may well have been limited by the brevity of the project and by the age of the students when they were first reached. The fact that age at first intercourse was delayed at all is impressive, and particularly important in view of the demonstrated high risks of early exposure to pregnancy.

Similarly, the results indicating that students attended clinics sooner after initiating sexual activity than had been the case are important. The project appears to demonstrate that if students in junior high schools are given access to nearby services and if they are offered information and continuity of care, they will use such services, and at levels comparable to those shown by older teenagers. That was clearly the case in this demonstration project, where confidential services were provided free of cost and in a sympathetic setting. Furthermore, the percentage of students going to a clinic or doctor before their first intercourse increased, as did attendance during the first months of sexual activity. Both these measures of preventive behavior were low at the time of the baseline survey, as they were among clinic patients observed in an earlier study, and both increased markedly.

One of the most striking findings from the project is the demonstration that boys in the junior high school used the clinic as freely as girls of the same age. In view of the growing call for

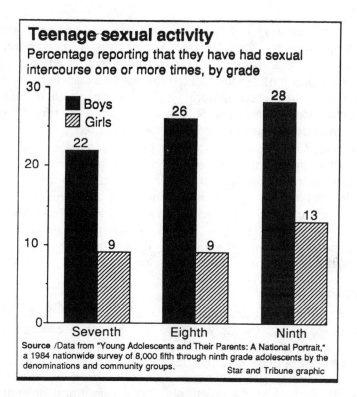

Teenage sexual activity

Percentage reporting that they have had sexual intercourse one or more times, by grade

- ■ Boys
- ▨ Girls

Seventh: Boys 22, Girls 9
Eighth: Boys 26, Girls 9
Ninth: Boys 28, Girls 13

Source /Data from "Young Adolescents and Their Parents: A National Portrait," a 1984 nationwide survey of 8,000 fifth through ninth grade adolescents by the denominations and community groups. Star and Tribune graphic

Reprinted by permission of the *Star Tribune,* Newspaper of the *Twin Cities.*

research into ways of attracting male clients to such facilities, the interest shown by these boys appears to be of some importance.

Behavior Change

The changes in contraceptive use demonstrated by the evaluation are promising. Again, the results among the younger students suggest that early risk of pregnancy can be reduced with early attendance at a clinic. Use of the condom did not change consistently, but appeared to fluctuate with the use of female methods in such a way that the overall use of all methods requiring advance preparation increased significantly.

Increased and prompt clinic attendance and the resulting increased use of effective methods of contraception appear to have had a significant impact on pregnancy levels. The full extent of this impact may not have been fully realized by the time follow-up was completed. Each of the measures we used confirms the finding of a reduction in pregnancy rates among older teenagers and a halt in the rapid increases—by some measures, a decrease—in the rates among younger adolescents. In the face of rising rates in many U.S. cities, the marked reduction in pregnancy demonstrated here is to be welcomed.

As successful as this program appears to have been, a longer period than that involved here is probably needed to achieve and to measure the full impact of interventions such as these. Many effects may not be quick in coming, and although our study reports many significant effects, one would hope that with time, even more young people might be affected. Perhaps the evidence we present will encourage the investment of funds and energies in similar programs, over a longer term.

Early Exposure

Furthermore, early program exposure is clearly of some importance; interventions will have to take place before young people develop behavior that places them at risk of early, postpubertal conception. The effects of this program apparently were somewhat greater among younger than among older students. One of its major effects, indeed, is that it appears to have encouraged the younger sexually active teenagers to develop levels of knowledge and patterns of behavior usually associated only with older adolescents. This accelerated protective behavior, coupled with evidence that first coitus was not encouraged but, in fact, postponed, should provide solid support to the current movement toward the introduction of school-based clinics. The model described here is a combined school and clinic operation that offers full reproductive health services and that is located close to, but not in, the school. When two schools are close enough to share a clinic, this may be a particularly economical model; further analysis of the component services may suggest an even more parsimonious design that could achieve many of the same results.

Conclusion

In conclusion, these findings suggest the efficacy of a program with pregnancy prevention as an explicit objective. Such a model requires a program and a staff capable of addressing a wide range of reproductive health issues. It does not preclude a broader range of adolescent health services (since these, too, are often badly needed), but it does suggest that meeting the sexual concerns, medical needs and contraceptive requirements of high school boys and girls is in itself an extremely challenging and demanding responsibility for program designers. More broad-based initiatives would, no doubt, have to include in their staffs some health educators, social workers, nurses or doctors with a strong commitment to the reproductive health of young people if they seek to replicate these results.

Why did this program work? Access to high-quality, free services was probably crucial to its success. Professional counseling, education and open communication were, no doubt, also important. All these factors appear to have created an atmosphere that allowed teenagers to translate their attitudes into constructive preventive behavior. Precisely which separate components of the program contributed most to its success remains to be determined. Our understanding of similar school-based services for young people may well depend on the willingness of providers to scrutinize their interventions closely, on the ability of researchers to evaluate those interventions and on the cooperation of schools in making available the types of data needed to carry out such evaluations.

14 PREVENTING TEENAGE PREGNANCY

REMOVING ADVERTISING RESTRICTIONS ON CONTRACEPTIVES

The Population Institute

The following statement was made by the Population Institute, 777 United Nations Plaza, New York, New York 10017.

Points to Consider

1. What has been the role of the courts?
2. How does the print media compare to television in advertising contraceptives?
3. Why is the right to know a cornerstone of American democracy?
4. Why is contraceptive information hidden from millions of youth by our society?
5. What arguments are advanced by the opponents of contraceptive information?

The Population Institute, "The Right to Know," United Nations, August, 1975.

In advertising, and particularly of nonprescription contraceptives, the answer in far too many instances has been an uncompromising no, a no which has led, we feel, to human heartbreak, social liabilities and economic upheaval.

The public has a "right to know", and advertising is one means to achieve such knowledge. Courts have stated that laws preventing the advertising of nonprescription contraceptives violate the public interest.

The public has a need to know about nonprescription contraceptives. There is no evidence to indicate that such knowledge leads to increased sexual activity, while a lack of knowledge does lead to unwanted children and abortion.

Contraceptive Products

A wide variety of contraceptive products are available. Individuals should be given the opportunity to choose among them based on informed judgment and personal requirements.

The provision of information about contraception is so important to society that all forms of media bear responsibility for its dissemination.

In so doing, the media will only be conforming to changed social attitudes. These enlightened attitudes are evidenced by public opinion polls; the positions of religious, medical and social organizations; court opinions; and government programs.

Already, the print media in this country are increasingly open to nonprescription contraceptive advertising. Worldwide, both print and broadcast media are even more receptive to such advertising.

The time is now appropriate for those in authority in the media to permit the advertising of nonprescription contraceptives.

A Cornerstone

The *right to know* is a fundamental cornerstone of American democracy. It is written into our Constitution; it is the basic tenet of our free press; it is the source of much of the vigor of our institutions; and from it issues much of the progress of our society, our culture and our industry.

Advertising is one avenue through which much information is conveyed to the public—not just product or service information but "information of potential interest and value to a diverse audience" as well.

When state or federal laws operate to ban " 'public interest' and mixed, as well as purely commercial advertising and display", they run "afoul of the Constitution".

The quotations cited above are from [1] the U.S. Supreme Court (Bigelow vs. Virginia) and [2] the U.S. District Court, Southern District of New York (Population Services International, et al., vs. Malcolm Wilson, et al.).

Both cases bear on the public's right to know. The first [1] voids a Virginia statute banning the advertising of abortion services. The second [2] declares unconstitutional the New York State law banning the sale, display and advertising of non-prescription contraceptives. In both cases federal courts declared that to prevent such advertising was to violate the interest of the public.

The Press

In the United States the press has tenaciously clung to its right to convey to the public what is its right to know. Radio and television are licensed by the federal government to operate in behalf of "the public interest, convenience and necessity".

It is a matter of grave public concern that at a time when the courts are striking down statutes banning the public's right to know via advertising having to do with the matters of contraception, pregnancy and abortion, the leaders of much of the mass media are effectively prohibiting such advertising through their institutional regulations and prohibitions.

The media have understandably raised the question of these subjects' "fitness" for the general audience. Editorially, the answer has generally been a confident yes. But in advertising, and particularly of nonprescription contraceptives, the answer in far too many instances has been an uncompromising no, a no which has led, we feel, to human heartbreak, social liabilities and economic upheaval. Each unwanted pregnancy serves as a sad judgment upon a society in which information and services regarding responsible sexuality are withheld from those in greatest need.

Sexual Responsibility

"We're saying, 'Let's have some balance,'" insists Planned Parenthood president Faye Wattleton. Real balance means lowering the random sexual content of programs while raising the times people act and talk responsibly.

In the daytime world of soaps, 94 percent of the sexual encounters are between people not married to each other. They do not stop to ask: Are you protected?

Another place to seek balance is in the commercials. Network advertisers are encouraged to use sex to sell everything . . . except birth control. The only contraceptives sold on network TV are for "birth control for roaches" . . .

"They tell us," says Wattleton, "that they don't want to offend the sensitivity of their viewers because birth control is controversial." Rape, murder, mayhem and menage a trois are apparently inoffensive. But even though 90 percent of adult Americans use contraceptives, they are labeled "controversial."

Ellen Goodman, *Boston Globe,* 1986

Though family planning—the right and ability of individuals and couples to regulate the number and spacing of their children—is now an accepted, legitimate social concept, it is, like so many other ideas which have won broad agreement and easy lip service, far from fulfillment. The sad reality remains that many women in this country still experience the tragedy of unwanted births. Too many babies are born unwanted—and uncared for. Many young careers and hopes are dashed by too-early parenthood . . .

Unwanted Pregnancy

A generation ago unwanted pregnancy was only whispered about. We all knew of stunned and heartbroken girls shunted into hiding for their pregnancies. Some were later able to put their broken lives back together, scars and all, but many others never could. Now we are slightly more enlightened. Some stigmas have lessened, yet many strictures remain. Among a large share of predominantly middle-aged decision-makers, sex and contraception openly discussed are embarrassing. The patterns of their own adolescence are still operative and these subjects are best relegated to locker rooms. The tragic consequences of these attitudes are visited every year on many hundreds of thousands of women and girls.

In our society, sex education and contraceptive information are "no-nos" for millions of youth and former youth. Yet admission to adulthood for a girl is pregnancy, at which point sex education and contraceptive counseling and products become available. Then too she can have an abortion, put her baby up for adoption, or become a prematurely aging teen mother . . .

It is generally recognized that venereal disease has become a widespread and serious epidemic. This realization has helped to ease strictures and create a necessary public dialogue in many forums, including the mass media. What is not realized is that adolescent pregnancy may be much more widespread . . .

Contraceptive Knowledge and Sexual Activity

Opponents of unlimited contraceptive information sometimes advance the argument that such freedom will inevitably result in increased sexual activity among unmarried persons, especially the young. If contraceptives are freely advertised, they say, young people will assume this indicates social approval and thus tend to encourage sexual activity. The fact is that there is already a significant incidence of coital activity among America's teenagers . . .

There is little evidence from the data on U.S. family planning programs which serve young people that the programs themselves have been responsible for raising the level of sexual activity. A recent study of such programs in Los Angeles showed that 96% of the 502 patients attending clinics were *already* sexually active by the time they came to the clinic,* suggesting

---

* Of these 482, only 186 had ever used any kind of contraceptive. Of the 186, 44% had relied upon condoms.

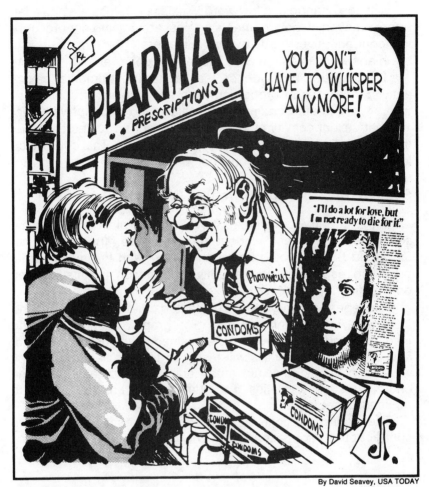

that the prospect of youngsters seeking contraceptive information and services in order to find out more about sex, or to prepare for initiation into sexual activity, is a myth.

The courts have spoken on this issue. In Population Services International vs. Malcolm Wilson, the State of New York claimed that it had "an interest in promoting the morality of its young people by seeking to discourage promiscuity and extramarital sexual intercourse. . . . Were contraceptives made available to minors . . . the State would seem to be sanctioning sexual activity by its young persons and thereby encouraging promiscuity".

With the change of a few words in these quotes, one has a fair approximation of the arguments against advertising nonprescription contraceptives made by media leaders.

In answer to this argument, the federal court replied: "We note . . . that 'there is no evidence that teenage extramarital sexual activity increases in proportion to the availability of contraceptives'. . . . [C]areful scrutiny . . . reveals . . . no evidence whatever . . . that sexual activity among young persons . . . decreases as the availability of contraceptives is restricted". The court ruled legal restrictions to be unconstitutional.

Some of the Costs of Unwanted Children

In this country, government-funded family planning programs serve needy women. Without this resource, the number of unwanted babies would be much larger. With the mass media providing responsible contraceptive information, this statistic can be significantly reduced.

The repercussions of these unwanted children go well beyond statistics. Any psychiatrist can give graphic testimony to the emotional and spiritual damage sustained by the unwanted child. Law enforcement officers will testify to the problems posed by youth and adults who, unwanted and deprived, have become enormous social liabilities. The human costs are so large as to be unassessable . . .

The economic cost of depriving Americans of access to contraceptive information and services is very large indeed.

PREVENTING TEENAGE PREGNANCY

CONTRACEPTIVE COMMERCIALS ARE INAPPROPRIATE

Alfred R. Schneider

Alfred R. Schneider is Vice President for Policy and Standards of Capital Cities/ABC, Inc. The Department of Standards and Practices, which reviews all entertainment programming and commercials prior to broadcast, reports to him.

Points to Consider

1. What is the objective of network programming?
2. Why do some viewers object to contraceptive advertising?
3. What is the responsibility of the local station?
4. How do network policies toward advertising and programming differ?
5. How should the AIDS crisis affect the advertising of condoms?

Excerpted from testimony by Alfred R. Schneider before the Subcommittee on Health and the Environment of the House Committee on Energy and Commerce, February 10, 1987.

A significant portion of our viewers feel contraceptive commercials are inappropriate or offensive, because they appear within or adjacent to programs that they may be viewing with their families, and these commercials appear without warning and out of context.

One of my responsibilities is to ensure that ABC Television Network's programming and commercials meet standards of good taste and community acceptability. We undertake this task because of the special nature of broadcast television, which is an invitee into millions of viewers' homes.

Unlike a newspaper, book or a magazine or cable television, where an affirmative decision to purchase is involved, we are present in 99 percent of American homes with television, instantly available to all at the flick of a switch.

Of all the communications media, television is the most personal, immediate and far reaching. Given the broad diversity of our national audience in age, education, social value and mores, broadcast television demands special care and responsibility. We pay careful attention to those needs, those wants and those concerns of our viewers, and attempt to be responsive by monitoring viewer reaction, analyzing public opinion research and holding meetings with a variety of special interest groups and organizations.

Our objective is to provide programming which is considered acceptable and appropriate by a diverse mainstream audience. This objective expands to our policy regarding the review and acceptance of advertising as well.

Contraceptive Advertising

The issue regarding acceptance of contraceptive advertising goes to the heart of these concerns. Such advertising clearly raises complex moral, ethical, and religious questions, which can be difficult to address or resolve satisfactorily in a 15 or 30 second commercial.

Furthermore, a significant portion of our viewers feel contraceptive commercials are inappropriate or offensive, because they appear within or adjacent to programs that they may be viewing with their families, and these commercials appear without warning

Condom Advertising

We note that there are currently 1227 commercial television stations in the United States. Yet by late last week, individual local television stations in only eleven markets had chosen to accept condom advertising. Their managements have made those decisions based on intimate knowledge of their own communities. It is reasonable to expect that other stations may elect to do the same—but only as their managements are secure in their assessment of attitudes in those communities. That is consistent with their obligations as licensees, their judgment as local business people and their sense of responsibility as professional broadcasters. For, as we all know, community standards and the extent of public health concerns vary greatly from locality to locality . . .

As a national broadcasting medium, we must obviously take into account all of these factors in considering an issue as uniquely sensitive as this. At the present time, we are not yet persuaded that a change in our network policy is indicated. However, the American public is clearly in the midst of an educational process and a reevaluation of attitudes with respect to the AIDS epidemic. I can assure you that we will be watching that process very closely as we continue to consider this issue.

George Dessart, Vice President, Program Practices, CBS News, Congressional Hearing, February 10, 1987

and out of context. These concerns have been the basis for our long standing policy against carrying such advertising on the ABC Television Network.

Let me stress that as we analyze these difficult and sensitive issues of commercial acceptance, we are required to play the role of surrogate for over 200 affiliated stations representing over 200 individual markets, markets with widely varying mores, attitudes and values.

In the final analysis, it is the local station licensee that makes the decision to carry any commercial or program. It is the local station that has the knowledge and understanding of the community it serves and it is the local station that is in the best position to determine what constitutes operating in the public interest, convenience and necessity on sensitive issues in its own community. Accordingly, we have treated the issue as an issue which rests with these local stations and local options. Until very recently, our affiliates have by and large concluded that they will not accept such advertisements.

Advertising and Programming

Before I turn to the very recent developments in the commercial acceptance area, let me state that our policies on contraceptive advertising do not apply to programming. Our entertainment, information and news programming have addressed the issues regarding contraception, sexuality and health concerns.

In that regard, let me specifically mention one program, a 2 hour made for television drama, tentatively entitled "Daddy," which is scheduled to appear on the ABC Television Network this coming Spring. The program will deal frankly with the issue of unintended teenage pregnancy and it discusses issues of sexual behavior, contraception and personal responsibility in a frank and candid manner.

The program is both realistic and relevant to teenagers and to adults who are naturally concerned about the social problem. We hope this is a program which will be viewed by both parents and their teenagers and that it will stimulate a discussion among parents and their children about issues surrounding teenage sexuality, within the context of a family's personal lives and personal values.

I am providing an attachment which details additional examples of broadcasts in 1986 and other years that are available, if you desire.

As we see it, the difference between programming and commercials is that programming offers the opportunity to discuss complex social moral concerns in depth and provides a context for doing so. Further, audiences can be made aware of the subject matter of the program and decide in advance whether or not to view them.

Commercials, on the other hand, offer neither the time, the context nor the possibility of advance warning to those who might not wish to watch such material.

AIDS Epidemic

The recent attention devoted to the AIDS epidemic has of course introduced a new concern. We have been asked to approve a broadcast for certain condom advertising which addresses the medical fact that the use of the condom may lower the risk of transmitting the AIDS virus.

Our position with respect to this issue is that while condoms may afford a measure of such protection against AIDS, it is impossible to separate this product use from the original and long standing use of the product, which is for birth control purposes.

Accordingly, acceptance of health related contraceptive advertisements for condoms necessarily means that we would soon be accepting a variety of contraceptive advertisements making a variety of product claims.

Nevertheless, as responsible broadcasters and as concerned citizens, we cannot fail to recognize the special responsibility which the AIDS problem may impose upon us. We are exploring whether we can develop and broadcast appropriate public service announcements with various agencies that consider the concerns I have outlined. We are paying close attention to the decisions being made by our affiliates and our own stations regarding the acceptance of condom advertisements.

As I have suggested, the local stations are, out of necessity, our weathervanes on issues such as this. We are and will be carefully reviewing and following their attitudes of all of American society with respect to this subject.

PREVENTING TEENAGE PREGNANCY

DECEIVING OURSELVES ABOUT SAFE SEX

Anthony B. Robinson

The following article by Anthony B. Robinson was taken from the Christian Century, *a liberal protestant ecumenical weekly magazine.*

Points to Consider

1. What different meanings can the term "safe sex" have?
2. How can safe sex be defined in terms of a workshop on AIDS?
3. How is the term "casual sex" defined?
4. What might the church have to say about sex?
5. How are the novelists defining sex?

What the church might say is that sex, no matter how we would like to kid ourselves into believing otherwise, is not safe, tidy, neat and risk-free, and it never will be. Sex is a gift and a mystery, something of which we are not fully in control, and which needs to be approached with some measure of awe and respect.

One evening several months ago when my wife returned from attending a planning meeting for an upcoming statewide church youth camp, I asked, as spouses are wont to do, how the meeting had gone. "OK, but . . ." she answered. She went on to explain that some of the planners had suggested a workshop on "safe sex." That had sounded good, she said—it was an important topic to raise with our junior-high-age kids. But as the discussion unfolded it became apparent that what was meant by a workshop on "safe sex" was instruction in how to use condoms in order to avoid AIDS. That approach may be appropriate for the public-health department, but for the church? Shouldn't the church have something more to say to its young people? Shouldn't the church have something to say about values, relationships, meaning?

Safe Sex

Time has passed and "safe sex" is the newly popular slogan. I have found myself wondering about this term. It seems the kind of technological jargon that contemporary society likes to kid itself into believing. We would like to think that sex is or can be safe, neat, tidy, without risk, without strings. We would like to think that sex is something that can be safely shut up in a little compartment of our busy lives. Thinking that we have so much else in our world under control, we would like to believe that sex too is under control. We're mightily disturbed that it's not.

This is not to say that we don't need complete information about AIDS and its prevention. And it's not to say that the church does not have a responsibility to minister to persons suffering from AIDS. But perhaps we also need to see our current situation as an opportunity to uncover some of the illusions and deceptions that our overly rationalistic and individualistic society has about sex and intimate relationships.

In reading fiction over the past year I have been struck by the number of authors who focus on some aspect of family life, or on intimate relationships, or on sex. Both male and female writers of our day are exploring the often bewildering and yet much-sought-after reality we designate, rather inadequately, as "family." Mary Gordon, Anne Tyler, Francine du Plessix Gray, Richard Ford, Thomas McGuane and John Updike are some of the contemporary authors exploring the mystery and brokenness of human and sexual relationships and of the family.

What these novelists are saying, in part, is that sex and intimacy are not a simple matter of momentary pleasure or an expression of autonomous individuals—which is what our technological, capitalist society would like to have us think. Sex and intimate relationships are, rather, as the ancients knew, full of mystery and power, of grace and danger. They are not something of which we are fully in control. They are not something that can be described as "safe" by anybody except the foolish or the fooled.

The Old Testament Hebrew phrase for sexual intercourse is "to know." Thus "Adam knew Eve." Perhaps this phrase is not so euphemistic as it seems. It suggests, at least, that when we are sexually involved with another, it is a *person* with whom we are involved. It suggests that, like it or not, intend it or not, something more than biological happens between two people who know each other sexually.

Writing about lust, ethicist William May describes the act of sexual intercourse as "the most intimate, complete, and unconditional unveiling of which two human beings are capable." He goes on to say that "as such, it is a gesture that is misleading and confusing whenever made in a context that is less than total self-giving." "Misleading" and "confusing" aptly describe a good deal of contemporary sexual behavior.

Casual Sex

The point of these observations is that casual sex is not simply wrong in itself but problematic because of the mixed messages it conveys. People get confused and become distrustful in a society where an act which says "I give myself" does not mean that at all. Community is undermined by this kind of mixed message.

110

Sexuality and the Media

- *The average American family has a television set turned on over seven hours each day.*
- *Teenagers watch approximately 24 hours of TV each week.*
- *Adolescents, aged 12 to 17 years old, listen to the radio approximately 18.5 hours each week.*
- *There are approximately 20,000 scenes of suggested sexual intercourse and behavior, sexual comment, and innuendo in a year of prime-time television.*
- *Television portrays six times more extramarital sex than sex between spouses. Ninety-four percent of the sexual encounters on soap operas are between people not married to each other.*

"The Facts," *Center for Population Options,* 1986

Stanley Hauerwas has criticized the liberal churches for being "public legalists and private antinomians." We pronounce on issues of national policy with great certainty, but when it comes to bedroom policy we seem to have little to say. An unequivocal embrace of the "safe sex" slogan may be only the latest illustration of the relevance of Hauerwas's critique.

In my town we've lately been treated to something called "the theology of condoms" by a local ecumenical leader. He has urged the church to talk about condoms. Well, yes, we want to protect ourselves and our children, but doesn't everybody? Who needs the church to say that?

What the church might say is that sex, no matter how we would like to kid ourselves into believing otherwise, is not safe, tidy, neat and risk-free, and it never will be. Sex is a gift and a mystery, something of which we are not fully in control, and which needs to be approached with some measure of awe and respect. Sexual activity has many consequences, and sex is a gift that entails responsibility. In proclaiming this message we will not solve all our problems, but at least we will not deceive our children and ourselves.

INTERPRETING EDITORIAL CARTOONS

This activity may be used as an individualized study guide for students in libraries and resource centers or as a discussion catalyst in small group and classroom discussions.

Although cartoons are usually humorous, the main intent of most political cartoonists is not to entertain. Cartoons express serious social comment about important issues. Using graphic and visual arts, the cartoonist expresses opinions and attitudes. By employing an entertaining and often light-hearted visual format, cartoonists may have as much or more impact on national and world issues as editorial and syndicated columnists.

Points to Consider

1. Examine the cartoon in this activity. (see next page)
2. How would you describe the message of the cartoon? Try to describe the message in one to three sentences.
3. Do you agree with the message expressed in the cartoon? Why or why not?
4. Does the cartoon support the author's point of view in any of the readings in this publication? If the answer is yes, be specific about which reading or readings and why.
5. Are any of the readings in chapter two in basic agreement with the cartoon?

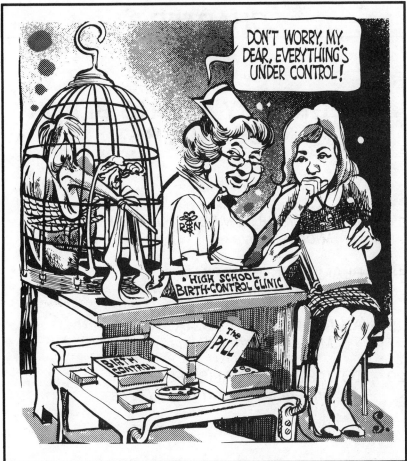

By David Seavey, USA TODAY

Copyright *USA Today*. Reprinted with permission.

CHAPTER 3

PREGNANCY AMONG BLACK TEENAGERS

17   THE VANISHING MALE CHARACTER
      Michael Novak

18   BLAMING THE VICTIM
      Chris Booker

19   AN AGENDA FOR SOCIAL REFORM
      Marian Wright Edelman

20   TOWARD A SOCIALIST FUTURE
      Angela Davis and Fania Davis

PREGNANCY AMONG BLACK TEENAGERS

THE VANISHING MALE CHARACTER

Michael Novak

Michael Novak is a Catholic theologian and works in religion and public policy at the American Enterprise Institute, a conservative "think tank" that attempts to influence public policy. He is a co-founder of Crisis *magazine, a conservative journal of lay Catholic opinion and a frequent contributor to the* National Review *magazine.*

Points to Consider

1. Why was the TV documentary by Bill Moyers a courageous statement?
2. What is meant by the vanishing male character?
3. How many black children are born out of wedlock?
4. Who was Timothy and what was his attitude?
5. What role is government playing in the problems of the black family?

Michael Novak, "The Content of Their Character," *National Review,* February 26, 1986, p. 47. © by the *National Review,* Inc., 150 East 35 Street, New York, NY 10016. Reprinted with permission.

Since there is no basic alternative except the family for character formation, the vanishing of the black family raises what Harvard's Glenn C. Loury calls "The Moral Quandary of the Black Community."

Martin Luther King, Jr. had a dream—that one day "Negro children will be judged not by the color of their skin but by the content of their character." Today, at last, that dream is coming true, but the judgment is far from what King would have wished.

Vanishing Family

According to one of the bravest TV documentaries ever made, by Bill Moyers of CBS (January 25), there is a crisis in black America: *The Vanishing Family*. Behind the gruesome statistics lies a deeper story: the vanishing of male character. Only a tiny fraction of black children born in America has a father at home during all 16 years of childhood. Nearly 60 per cent are born out of wedlock. Such matriarchy is proving colossally destructive.

Since there is no basic alternative except the family for character formation, the vanishing of the black family raises what Harvard's Glenn C. Loury calls "The Moral Quandary of the Black Community." Dare one call attention to this sinking, *Titanic*-like underclass culture? Dare one not?

Thanks to the courage of Bill Moyers, the CBS documentary introduces us to some immensely attractive young women and young men in Newark's black ghetto. How bright and alive they seem, yet how ineffably sad.

Timothy

Timothy, for example, is 26, handsome, and —he says quite truthfully—attractive to women; he has had six children by four different girls. It doesn't bother him that he doesn't support them. (They may, in fact, be supporting him.) "Well, the majority of the mothers are on welfare. . . . What I'm not doing, the government does."

Winsome and pregnant with her third child, his girl Alice poignantly adds: "I don't think I would have had the second two children if I didn't think welfare was there. I don't like welfare because it makes me lazy. . . . Yeah, it makes you lazy just to sit

Sexual Recklessness

Today nearly 60 percent of all black children are born out of wedlock. Imagine the astronomic percentages in many inner cities. Black girls between ages 15 and 19 are the most fertile population of that age group in the industrialized world. Half of all black teenage girls become pregnant. The resulting "families" rarely are self-supporting. Almost half of all black children are partially supported by government payments . . .

Young blacks, whose sexual recklessness produces oceans of misery, feel little of the kind of guilt that changes behavior. One reason for this is that they have been taught by reflexive "civil rights" rhetoric that they are mere victims, absolved from responsibility by the all-purpose alibi of "white racism."

George F. Will, *The Washington Post*, January, 1986

around and wait for a monthly check to come in. You know, I just like to work. I like having money coming in every week or every two weeks." On "mothers' day," once each month, the mothers of her area gather to collect the money.

Come in it does. Alice receives $385 a month, plus $112 in food stamps. If each of Timothy's other girls does as well, that means some $2,000 per month for the four girls. Witnessing Alice's delivery of her third child, Timothy shouts: "I'm a king!"

"That's all they be doing around here," Darren Lyell, 18, says, concerning his male friends. "Making babies and stuff. Making babies." His daughter was born to Clarinda, 15, who says: "I wouldn't want no man holding me down, because I think I could make it as a single parent." Her mother did. Her grandmother, too.

One admires tremendously these brave but lonely young women, who are invariably well dressed; the rooms they live in boast an admirable range of appliances. "They are married to welfare," another youngster says. The government is the father.

Brutality

The lives their young black men live are staggering in their brutality. One tells Moyers how he tied metal to a baseball bat and went seeking some young men who had insulted him and "got even." Many bear scars from beatings and knife play. One in 15 will be murdered by age twenty-five.

George Gilder described all this several years ago in *The Visible Man,* a book little reviewed, little purchased. The story Moyers told on television repeated several themes noted by Gilder: the trip back to North Carolina in which one could see ancient family strengths and a powerful sense of religion; the raw artistic talent of one of the willfully unemployed protagonists.

Carolyn Wallace, a magnificent social worker in Newark, tells Moyers that people today don't want to hear about "morality" and "God," but they must, for the problem is not a government problem, but a moral problem. We have to keep saying that, she says. She tells Moyers: "If you say it in your corner and I say it in my corner, and everybody's saying it, it's going to be like a drumbeat." Back to basics. Back to character.

Government *is* in the morality business today—an immoral morality. Television entertainment and the movies are also in the morality business—an immoral morality. Newark police detective Shahid Jackson, a true moral hero, can afford no illusions: "When I was growing up, sex was a dirty word. Now sex is what's happening. You know, they see sex on TV, sex in the movies, sex everywhere.

It isn't sex that is dirty. But fatherhood that ends with the sex act means treating male responsibilities like dirt. One does not admire—and youngsters must know that adults do *not* admire —the content of such a character.

Poor Kids

If these are poor kids, they certainly don't look, dress, or act poor; rather, like spoiled children of the rich. They have a sugar daddy. His name is Uncle Sam.

Among our elites, James Q. Wilson writes in a recent issue of *The Public Interest,* modernity means "replacing the ethic of self-control with that of self-expression." One does not see much self-control in these Newark streets; one sees much self-expression. Just as on television.

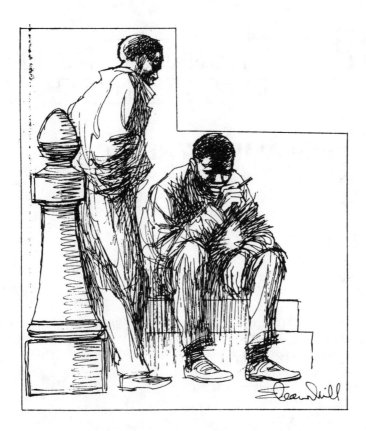

It is wrong to do this to poor kids, morally wrong, socially wrong, politically wrong, economically wrong. We need, indeed, a second War on Poverty. This time, though, it must have a moral focus. This drumbeat must start in every corner of the land: *It is shameless, immoral, and unmanly for fathers to abandon their children.* Man-children need to be helped by everyone's holding them to that.

PREGNANCY AMONG
BLACK TEENAGERS

BLAMING THE VICTIM

Chris Booker

Chris Booker wrote the following comments in the Guardian, *a weekly tabloid newspaper presenting radical views on social and political issues.*

Points to Consider

1. How is the Bill Moyers' TV program titled "The Vanishing Family" described?
2. What were the central themes of the Moyers program?
3. Who was Timothy and how was he described?
4. What was the Moynihan Report?
5. How did the black community react to the Moyers program?

Chris Booker, "Blame the Victim, Not Racism, Says CBS," *Guardian,* February 19, 1986, p. 20.

There is a broad agreement in the Black community that the high rate of teen pregnancy is a problem. But to look at the issue, as Moyers did, separated from the realities of institutional racism and poverty helps no one.

Recent months have witnessed an upsurge in reports attributing the growing social crises in Black communities to the victims themselves. The chorus of voices pointing the finger of blame at the Black impoverished reached a new peak with the airing of Bill Moyers's "The Vanishing Family." Using interviews with fewer than 10 low-income Blacks, Moyers hammered home a few central themes: Blacks themselves, not racism, are their own worse enemy; welfare is destroying the fabric of the Black family; Black men are generally irresponsible; Black youth are increasingly immersed in a culture of violence, rampant sexual excess and dependence on government "handouts."

Atypical Youth

Much of the show's focus is on quite atypical Black youth. Timothy, 26, flattered by the sudden attention and clearly performing before the camera, glows with pride describing himself as "highly sexed." His light-hearted attitude toward his responsibilities as a father and his lack of concern since "welfare" will take care of his children are highlighted.

Portrayed as the typical Black young male, this father of six hasn't had a job in two-and-a-half years and has been arrested on robbery and drug charges.

Crowds gathering on the grounds of a Newark, N.J., housing project waiting for their welfare checks are shown. Moyers is told that the day the checks come is referred to as "Mother's Day," as if it were a holiday. The compelling evidence that welfare corrupts is provided by the welfare recipients themselves, whom Moyers quotes saying welfare makes them feel "lazy." A Black detective is prodded by Moyers to say that many Black men are living off the women's welfare checks, too. How below-subsistence welfare checks can be stretched to this extent is left unexplained.

Bill Moyers

Moyers's interest in the Black family is not new. During the mid-1960s he helped direct President Lyndon Johnson's attention to the Moynihan Report, which contended that at "the heart of the deterioration of the fabric of Negro society is the deterioration of the Negro family. It is the fundamental source of weakness of the Negro community at the present time. . . . Unless this damage is repaired, all the effort to end discrimination and poverty and injustice will come to little." This conclusion was widely condemned by Black activists as racist.

Moyers backs up the comments of the Black poor themselves with "experts" who agree with him. George Jackson, a Harvard University psychologist, says the problem is that their "values" don't properly constrain their behavior. Carolyn Wallace, a middle-class Black, says "racism is not the problem. . . . Society has made living easy." Wallace goes on to say, "We're destroying ourselves."

Fortunately, Moyers added a final 45-minute discussion which featured, among others, Jesse Jackson and Eleanor Holmes Norton. Norton noted that it was necessary to mobilize the Black community to confront the problems of teen pregnancy but she criticized the "cynical" notion that government was unable to contribute to their solution. Jesse Jackson called for a "massive counter-culture movement" against negative cultural practices within the Black community.

Some observers have used the Moyers documentary to focus their fire on the low-income Black community in particular, and the entire Black population in general. Syndicated columnist George Will, for instance, wrote that "young Blacks, whose sexual recklessness produces oceans of misery, feel little of the kind of guilt that changes behavior. One reason for this is that they have been taught by reflexive 'civil rights' rhetoric that they are mere victims, absolved from responsibility by the all-purpose alibi of 'white racism.' "

The Black Community

The nation's Black communities are clearly divided in their opinion of the Moyers documentary. At one extreme is conservative columnist Tony Brown, who believes Moyers didn't go far enough, and calls for punitive action—including imprisonment —against youth such as Timothy who don't support their

Black Female-Headed Families

The changing economic status of black Americans may be seen as a dual phenomenon. The poverty rate among black families consisting of a married couple (with or without children) dropped from more than 50 percent in 1959 to 14 percent in 1984, but the poverty rate among black female-headed families fell only from 70 to 52 percent during that period. Similarly, since 1968, the median income for black families headed by a married couple has risen 17 percent (in constant dollars), whereas the median income for black female-headed families has fallen by eight percent. This polarization can be seen most clearly in the changing structure of the population living in poverty. In 1959, fewer than 30 percent of all blacks in poverty lived in female-headed families; today, 68 percent of all poor blacks live in such families.

Tom Joe, *Family Planning Perspectives,* March/April, 1987

offspring. For the young women, he advocates penalizing cuts in the welfare payments and the establishment of special dormitories.

Councilman Donald Tucker of Newark, N.J., where the documentary was shot, was highly critical of the production. While the "portrayal of young Black men as mindless, irresponsible, moral degenerates may very well be true of the persons interviewed," he said, "it is not true of the majority of Black teenagers." The show "only serves to reinforce existing negative stereotypes of Black people by some viewers."

Kemba Maish, a clinical psychologist and community activist in Washington, D.C., housing projects, said that Moyers seemed to be trying to lead people to say "get rid of welfare." She criticized the documentary for neglecting to mention factors like drugs, unemployment and Black youths' low self-esteem, concluding that Moyers was reviving Moynihan's "blaming the victim" theory of Black oppression.

Marian Wright Edelman, president of the Children's Defense Fund, pointed to the same danger. She added that the reason

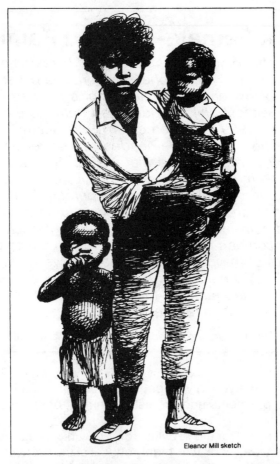

Eleanor Mill sketch

teen pregnancy is a problem now is "we no longer live in an America in which 18- and 19-year-old men can earn enough money to support a family, and because we never had an America in which the average single woman with children could earn a decent wage at any age." Youth should be taught, according to Edelman, "that early sexual activity, pregnancy and parenthood are undesirable." However, she stressed that this must be supported by some "payoff" in better education and employment opportunities if this effort is to be successful.

There is a broad agreement in the Black community that the high rate of teen pregnancy is a problem—and one that the community itself must confront and seek solutions to. But to look at the issue, as Moyers did, separated from the realities of institutional racism and poverty helps no one.

124

19 PREGNANCY AMONG BLACK TEENAGERS

AN AGENDA FOR SOCIAL REFORM

Marian Wright Edelman

Marian Wright Edelman is the president of the Children's Defense Fund.

Points to Consider

1. What role should all levels of government play to help solve the problem of teen pregnancy?
2. How can people and organizations outside government help?
3. Each year how many infants do teenagers give birth to?
4. What role does poverty play in the problem of teen pregnancy?

Excerpted from testimony by Marian Wright Edelman before the House Committee on Ways and Means, February 18, 1986.

As teenagers grow up and become sexually active, expectations and responsibility are linked closely. Disadvantaged children who are denied the hope, much less the expectation, that hard work will bring tangible rewards or that tomorrow can be better than today also have no motivation to learn to take responsibility for their futures.

There is no single cause of or group affected by adolescent pregnancy. Changes in our families, our values, and our economy all have contributed to the tragedy of children having children. And just as there is no one reason for teen pregnancies, there is no "quick fix"—no single solution that offers a complete or adequate response to this complex problem.

The proposals that follow—an agenda designed to prevent pregnancies and to help more of our young people become self-sufficient adults—represent only a first and a partial answer to the challenge of adolescent pregnancy prevention. They constitute an agenda for government—federal, state, and local.

Of course, government alone cannot solve this problem. To combat teen pregnancy in our communities, this agenda must be accompanied by our personal efforts—as parents and concerned citizens—to speak out and reach out to young people who are at risk of becoming teen parents. Through our families and our churches we must fight against the erosion of our children's values by the messages of the media, and work to reinstill a sense of personal responsibility and self-esteem among our youths. As leaders in our communities, we must provide strong and positive role models for our children, teaching by example the importance of self-help, compassion, and hard work. An agenda for parents and community organizations and institutions is set out in a separate Children's Defense Fund publication, "Preventing Children Having Children: What YOU Can Do."

Government Role

But government has an important role in helping to solve the problem. And this role goes beyond simply helping provide sex education or family planning services for sexually active teens, because the problem goes well beyond the absence of such education and services.

126

New Campaign Against Teen Pregnancy

Most parents hope their adolescent children will forgo sex until they're mature. But millions of teens ignore that wish; more than 1 million teenaged girls become pregnant every year. Thus parents should welcome the Children's Defense Fund's new campaign to reduce the teen birth rate. Launched last week in Minneapolis and seven other cities, the campaign's goal is to help parents and children face the reality of teenage sexual activity and to avoid the tragedy it spawns.

Minneapolis Star and Tribune, March 5, 1986

Too many of our young people today lack either the capacity or the motivation to delay pregnancy. It is true that without knowledge of the potential consequences of sexual activity and access to services that help prevent pregnancy, many teenagers unintentionally begin families before they are prepared to care for them. Of equal importance, however, too many of America's poor and minority youths who have no hopes for better futures become parents too young because they do not think that they have anything to lose. If they postpone parenthood, they believe, it will not help them finish school, or get a good education while in school, or get a decent job when they leave school. And too often this belief is correct.

The Agenda

For these reasons, the adolescent pregnancy prevention and youth self-sufficiency agenda calls for investments in our young people that will enable them not only to make responsible decisions but to move along a steady path toward self-sufficiency. The agenda reflects the need for progress on many fronts, addressing four basic goals: restoring hope and responsibility among youths, strengthening families, building a solid foundation for teenagers, and helping adolescents with special needs.

As teenagers grow up and become sexually active, expectations and responsibility are linked closely. Disadvantaged children who are denied the hope, much less the expectation, that hard work will bring tangible rewards or that tomorrow can be better than today also have no motivation to learn to take responsibility for their futures. The agenda includes innovative strategies for bolstering responsibility and hope, expanding opportunities for work and learning while also strengthening decisionmaking skills, rewarding hard work, and encouraging responsible behavior.

An adolescent pregnancy prevention strategy almost must provide teens the capacity to avoid pregnancy, both by making their families stronger and by supplying them with the services they need to avoid pregnancy. The agenda proposes essential improvements in health care, education, and other services for those adolescents at risk of becoming parents too young.

Finally, the agenda addresses the special needs of troubled adolescents and youths in out-of-home care who represent an especially vulnerable population. The agenda seeks to ensure that the futures of these young people are not further clouded by too-early parenthood.

Co-operative Effort

All levels of government—federal, state, and local—must tackle the problem of adolescent pregnancy and the challenge of helping youths grow into self-sufficient adults. Virtually every item on the agenda provides the basis of a pregnancy prevention initiative at each level of government. A teen health clinic will need federal and state funds as well as assistance from the city or county health department. School boards have a critical role to play, but they will need help from other levels of government to do the job fully. Given the magnitude of the task, the combined resources of federal, state, and local governments will be needed to mount an effective response. But no level of government should wait for the others to act first.

Some components of the agenda require immediate public investments in health care, child care, education, and income supports, investments which in the long term will yield important savings in government expenditures. Other elements can be implemented by reorganizing or improving existing services without additional resources or with minimal expense. Yet other

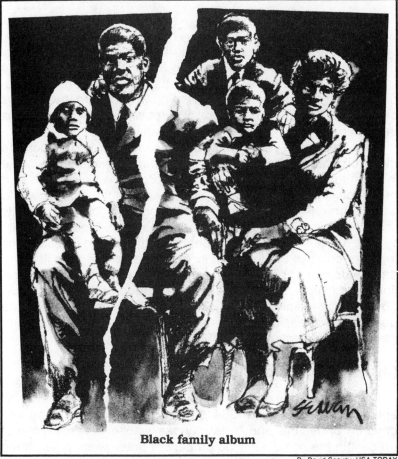

Black family album

By David Seavey, USA TODAY

elements, such as child support enforcement, should return more money than they cost, even in the short term.

In all cases, the long-range costs of inaction—human, social, and economic—warrant strong preventive measures to combat adolescent pregnancy.

A section-by-section summary of the adolescent pregnancy prevention and youth self-sufficiency agenda follows. For more information, contact CDF's Adolescent Pregnancy Prevention Clearinghouse.

Youth Opportunity Accounts

For many poor and minority youths, the future holds little promise. Those living in communities with few jobs or opportunities to develop their skills often find little reason to delay pregnancy and parenthood. Lacking a real chance to contribute to society and help themselves through work or service, disadvantaged teenagers often have no way to learn the rewards of sustained effort or the responsibilities and mutual obligations that are part of being a parent and an adult.

The creation of youth opportunity accounts would respond to these urgent needs by offering participating teenagers a stake in the future and an opportunity to improve their own skills and prospects through hard work and achievement. Youths would accrue credits in their opportunity accounts by successfully completing various education, work experience, and community service activities. They could subsequently redeem these credits to cover costs of participation in vocational training, postsecondary education, or paid employment opportunities. Demonstration efforts should be undertaken by the federal, state, and local governments—limited initially to a small number of sites—to document the feasibility of this approach and explore options for its broader implementation. . . .

Child Support Enforcement

Failure of absent parents to support their children has reached epidemic proportions. In 1984, 8.7 million women were living with children under the age of twenty-one whose fathers were not present in the home. Only 58 percent of these women had been awarded child support. Of those who were supposed to receive child support in 1983, only half received the amount due. Twenty-six percent received partial payment, and 24 percent received no payment at all.

States must undertake more rigorous efforts to establish child support obligations and to make child support collections on behalf of families seeking such services from the states . . .

After-School Care for Young Adolescents

In a recent poll conducted by the Center for Early Adolescence, parents of ten- to fifteen-year-old children said that they were unsure of their young adolescent children's needs, fearful for the well-being of their children, and bewildered about what to do to improve the situation. Young adolescents are also at risk when left for long hours in unsupervised settings. Young teenagers may become pregnant, or get involved in drug and alcohol abuse or juvenile delinquency . . .

Federal, state, and local funds must be provided for after-school programs for young adolescents. Legislative initiatives should provide authorization and funding to help communities start and operate a variety of programs that could be run by agencies ranging from schools to churches and community-based organizations. Community organizations also should explore the extent to which they can, within existing budgets, begin to develop after-school services in the interim.

Community Learning Centers

By the time they reach high school, some youths have established a pattern of academic failure in traditional classroom settings. The cycle of poor academic performance, low expectations, and eventual resignation can take hold even in junior high and middle schools, particularly among children who do not receive strong parental support for academic achievement or whose families don't have the resources to give them the help they need outside of school . . .

The development of community learning centers would build upon the strong record of existing remedial education programs operated by some community-based organizations to serve out-of-school youths and adults who lack basic academic skills, promoting literacy and GED preparation. Separate part-time programs would encourage and reinforce academic gains for youths still in school. Providing these services during after-school and weekend hours, the centers would supplement the efforts of public schools and strengthen the awareness of at-risk youths that basic skills are essential to future self-sufficiency.

Dropout Prevention

Young people who fail to finish high school are at substantially greater risk of becoming parents at an early age. They also are considerably less likely than their peers to become self-sufficient adults. High school dropouts are almost twice as likely as graduates to be unemployed. Research suggests that school completion is one of the most important factors influencing youths' future employment, earnings, and capacity for self-support . . .

This dropout initiative, which should receive federal, state, and local support and resources, would target funds to schools with high dropout rates for the development of community-based dropout prevention efforts . . .

A federal dropout prevention initiative should combine financial support for school improvement efforts with the creation of a nationwide data collection system to provide reliable information on school dropouts . . .

Jobs for Unemployed Youths

Today's youth unemployment rates, particularly among poor and minority teenagers, are unacceptably high. A paying part-time job can provide a powerful incentive to stay in school and also can build a base of work experience, enhancing future employability. The income, responsibility, hope, and self-esteem associated with paid employment strengthen the incentives and the motivation among teens to avoid early parenthood.

Direct job creation efforts, targeted at low-income youths and tied to school attendance or participation in an alternative education program, can bolster both academic achievement and future self-sufficiency. Part-time employment during the school year as well as full-time jobs in the summer months, subsidized in part by the public sector, would alleviate the overwhelming joblessness now found in most poor communities. Requirements that participants continue academic work also would stress the importance of basic skills and the responsibilities that accompany participation in this program of self-help . . .

Life Planning and Sex Education

Today's children are growing up in a world far more complicated and demanding than it was even thirty years ago. Teens normally are expected to delay the traditional markers of adulthood—completion of education, entrance into the labor force, marriage, and family formation—in order to accommodate needs for increased education, career exploration, and training. At the same time, however, we are placing greater demands on teenagers. Decisions made at ages thirteen, fifteen, and seventeen often play a crucial role in determining our youths' adult success—decisions about high school completion, college or vocational training, careers, and most important, parenthood.

Too few teens are being offered sufficient adult guidance in making these important decisions. Even fewer are being given instruction in how to make good decisions, or sound information about the importance of doing so. Too many teens drift into decisions that they later regret . . .

Family Planning Clinics

The federal Title X program provides essential health, family planning, and health education services to more than 1 million young women and mothers each year. It is a key element in any concerned effort to prevent teen pregnancy. The program is both effective and cost-effective. In 1981 alone, family planning clinics prevented more than 800,000 unintended pregnancies. Studies have shown that the program yields savings of $1.80 for every dollar invested . . .

Comprehensive Health Clinics for Adolescents and Extension of Medicaid Eligibility

The special health and related problems that teenagers face make it particularly important that they have access to health care providers who are committed and trained to serve them. Poor children in general tend to be low utilizers of health care, but teenagers' lack of utilization of health services is particularly alarming. Children between the ages of eleven and twenty are less likely to see a physician during a year than any other portion of the U.S. population . . .

Health clinics providing specialized services to teenagers during the past decade have shown remarkable success in identifying previously undisclosed and untreated health problems, assisting children in making the transition into adulthood through counseling, referral, and other supportive services, and dealing with such serious problems as substance abuse and mental health problems. These specialized clinics, by making teens healthier, have shown a measurable impact on absenteeism, have generated feelings of growing self-sufficiency, and ultimately have improved the productivity of their patients. Moreover, the clinics are a key part of a strategy to reduce teen pregnancy. Studies show that through family planning counseling, prescriptions, and follow-up they have been markedly successful in reducing the rate of unintended first and repeat pregnancies . . .

Child Care Services for the Children of Teen Parents

Each year, teenagers give birth to more than 500,000 infants. About 300,000 of these young mothers have not completed high school. Without education or training they usually face the prospect of low-paying jobs at best and welfare at worst. Women who drop out of high school, have no previous work experience, and become heads of families by having children without getting married are more likely to be dependent on welfare for the long term. Pregnancy is the largest single reason for girls dropping out of school.

The lack of child care may be the most critical factor keeping teen mothers from returning to school. A 1978 nationwide study of 125 large cities identified the most significant unmet needs for teenage mothers and their babies as facilities, funds, and staff to provide infant care, the growing number of adult mothers who are now in the labor force and have very young children compounds the overall demand for infant care, further exacerbating the dearth of such services for teen parents.

Historically, if school systems responded to this problem at all, it was through special alternative schools designed to isolate the pregnant teenager and teach parenting skills. Even now, schools that offer child care programs often limit services to the duration of the school semester after birth, leaving young mothers to cope with the difficult problem of finding child care, without resources to pay for it, after a few short months.

To remedy these problems, state legislation authorizing effective child care programs for young mothers should support programs located in or within easy access to high schools.

Policymakers must recognize the difficulty of finding affordable child care and structure programs to meet the needs of a teen parent at least until her infant is past the toddler stage and she finishes high school. Parent education and counseling available to the general student body is another essential element of such a program. Such education can help a young mother understand the basics of child rearing, and impress upon other students the serious nature of parenthood. Federal, state, and local funds should support these child care services for teen parents.

20 PREGNANCY AMONG BLACK TEENAGERS

TOWARD A SOCIALIST FUTURE

Angela Davis and Fania Davis

Angela Davis is a member of the Central Committee of the Communist Party, USA, and a co-chairperson of the National Alliance Against Racist and Political Repression. Fania Davis is an attorney and rights activist in California.

Points to Consider

1. How many African-American families revolve around single women?
2. Why does this happen?
3. Why is teen pregnancy a symptom of economic conditions in the black community?
4. How do conservatives explain the rise in black teen pregnancy?
5. What role does military spending play?
6. How can the status of the black family be improved?

Angela Davis and Fania Davis, "The Black Family Under Reaganite Attack," *Daily World,* February 20, 1986, pp. 12–13 M.

However urgent a problem teen pregnancy may be, it is certainly not the root cause of the deteriorating economic status of the Black community.

Over the centuries following the forcible transplantion of African people in North America, children have represented something very special—the promise of freedom for an entire people. Even as Black people's efforts to hold onto and strengthen their family ties were cruelly assaulted, the family remained for generations an important cauldron of resistance, forging and preserving a vital legacy of collective struggle for freedom. Though grandmothers and grandfathers could not expect to free themselves from slavery or sharecropping or Mr. Charlie's kitchen, at least they could pass on the dream.

Today, however, in the era of Reaganism, the lives and future of those to whom the dream should be offered are in greater jeopardy than ever before. According to the most recent report of the Children's Defense Fund, Black children today, as compared to five years ago, are much more likely to be born into devastating conditions of poverty.

Yet, the administration's ideologues have mounted a campaign designed to convince the public—the Black community included—that these appalling conditions emanate directly from the breakdown of the Black family structure.

The current ideological blame-shifting which targets the Black family reflects a larger trend of singling out the family in general, falsely represented as an isolated, privatized area of social life, as the locus of dangerous dysfunction in the moral well-being of U.S. society.

It is pointed out that almost half of all African-American families revolve around single women and that 55% of Black babies are born to unmarried mothers—a substantial number of them under 20.

Emanating from the Reagan administration are arguments that this breakdown in the structure of the Black family has been promoted by the welfare system. Thus, an immediate solution would involve the reduction of government programs and the requiring of individuals on welfare to offer their labor to the state as well as the implementation of programs designed to apprehend absent fathers, compelling them to contribute to the support of their children.

Feminization of Poverty

The feminization of poverty, among Afro-Americans and the tens of millions of other similarly situated poor people of all racial or ethnic groups, is in fact not a family crisis but an economic crisis. "Fatherlessness," the pervasiveness of female-headed households among Afro-Americans, reflects the astronomically high levels of Black male unemployment, underemployment, imprisonment, drug addiction and mortality—consequences of the economic impotence among Black men in a racist and patriarchal society. Because sex discrimination in payrates and salaries allow working women to earn an average of only 60% of the wages earned by men, economic fatherlessness condemns most female-headed families to poverty, even when single mothers are employed. Furthermore, the assault on welfare supports, such as Aid to Families with Dependent Children (AFDC), absolutely insures the impoverishment of almost all unemployed single mothers and their children.

Muhammad I. Kenyatta, *Guardian,* June 4, 1986

Robert B. Carleson, Reagan's advisor for social policy development, has put forth arguments holding existing government social programs responsible for the increasing number of single parent, female-centered households. Moreover, he has asserted that the main problem is the failure in the Black community to form families.

Yet the statistical evidence demonstrates that the great majority of female-centered households are caused, not by women bearing children who have never entered into legal marriage partnerships, but by the breakup of married couple families.

Of the single women heading families, only one-fourth have never been married: 28.7% are married with an absent spouse, 22.2% are widowed and 21.9% are divorced. Would the withdrawal of welfare payments resurrect dead fathers, annul divorces or cause unemployed husbands to return to their wives and children? Would it make sex education available to teenagers and would it bring into being safe, effective and accessible contraceptive measures?

Teen Pregnancies

This last question has serious implications since the birth rate among single Black teenagers actually declined during the 1970s—a fact which clearly flies in the face of the prevailing belief that Black teenage girls are having more babies than ever before. What has caused a disproportionate number of births to unmarried teenagers is the even more rapid decline in the birth rate among older and married Black women. These groups are far more likely to rely on contraception and to have abortions —and indeed to become sterilized—than unmarried Black teenagers.

However urgent a problem teen pregnancy may be, it is certainly not the root cause of the deteriorating economic status of the Black community. On the contrary, it is a symptom of a deeply rooted structural crisis in the U.S. monopoly capitalist economy whose reverberations are being felt most painfully in the African-American community.

There is a direct correlation between the unprecedented rates of unemployment among Black teenagers and the rise in the birth rate among Black women under 20. Yet, the policy shapers for the Reagan administration continue to formulate the problem of teenage pregnancies in terms that by implication hold Black girls at least in part responsible for the depressed state of the Black community.

The conservative ideologues who express outrage about the accelerated rate of Black teenage pregnancy and the corresponding breakdown of the Black family call forth directly or by implication old historical distortions about Black women's—and men's—morality—or lack thereof. They accuse government welfare programs of having encouraged the ethical failures of the Black community.

While there are many destructive pressures exerted on Black families, such as the increasing lack of quality education available to young Black people, the proliferation of drugs and the

138

prevalence of other anti-social phenomena directly encouraged by the racist institutions of this country, the most devastating encumbrance is the pervasive joblessness, especially among young Black men and women.

Joblessness

Current observations on the Black family never fail to point out that in the two decades following 1960, the percentage of single Black women with children rose from about 21% to 47%. What is seldom noticed, however, is that during the same historical period the percentage of employed adult Black men plummeted from approximately 75% to 55%.

It is common knowledge that government census figures undercount the Black population, which means that probably less than half of African-American males in this country actually hold jobs. Official unemployment rates among Black teenagers project a 50% rate of joblessness. However, the reality is that less than 20% actually hold jobs. The rest are simply not counted as being a part of the labor force.

Moreover, to unemployment must be added underemployment, as well as underpaid jobs. According to the Children's Defense Fund annual report, if almost half of all Black children are poor (as compared to one in six white children) it is because the median family income of Black families is less than 60% of that of white families. Half of all Black families had incomes below $14,000 in 1983.

Exactly 20 years ago, the government report authored by Daniel Moynihan, entitled "The Negro Family: Case for National Action," had strategic implications which justified the withdrawal of government measures designed to counter the special racist edge of the social crisis leading to the permanent impoverishment of the Black community.

Today, official spokesmen are proposing that government programs designed to bring some relief to poor families be curtailed, ostensibly to revive a two-parent family structure in the Black community.

Just as the ulterior aim of the Moynihan Report was to provide a philosophical justification for the reversal of government policy to eradicate the causes of racism in U.S. society, the present strategy is designed to shore up the Reaganite posture of denying the existence of institutionalized forms of racism in the post-civil rights era.

Proposed Solutions

Moynihan, in the meantime, has put forth a reassessment of his original views. He now argues that precisely because of the current pervasiveness of single parent families of all backgrounds and the impoverishment of those families, the resulting problems should be attributed, not simply to Black people, but to the society as a whole.

While this modified description of the problem certainly represents an improvement, Moynihan admits that he is incapable of proposing anything other than piecemeal solutions . . .

However, if progress is to be made, employment and education opportunities must be readily available. And the fact is that the U.S. economy has been rapidly phasing out jobs traditionally held by Black people, thus shoving ever larger numbers of our people to the outer margins of the economic life of this country . . .

Military Connection

A dominant feature of the current aggregate structural crisis is the increasing militarization of the productive process. In the process of retooling the productive process in accordance with the dictates of the military-industrial complex, creating the means with which to produce untold billions of dollars in weapons, whose destructive potential is unprecedented, Black people are being literally robbed of jobs—at the rate of 1,300 jobs for each increase of $1 billion in the military budget (Bread Not Bombs).

The runaway U.S. military budget is at the heart of an economic "tangle of pathology"—to borrow Moynihan's terminology—currently causing the devastation of the Black community and the resulting structural problems within the Black family.

Since 1980, the military budget has literally doubled, as non-military programs have been slashed by almost $100 billion. From 1981–1985, military budgets have totalled $1.2 trillion and the Pentagon has proposed $2 trillion more for the next five years.

Since 1980, six million more people have fallen into the ranks of the poor. Twenty million are hungry, yet one million have been taken off the food stamp rolls altogether. While subsidized housing has been cut by 63% since 1981, homelessness is growing at an alarming rate. (The Women's Budget, WILPF, June 1985)

Given the historic decline and contraction of the contemporary capitalist economy, exacerbated in large part by the rapid militarization of the productive process, it is plain that conditions of mass unemployment and rising poverty in our communities will not go away unless a radical anti-monopoly program of jobs with peace is instituted . . .

A Socialist Future

Our families cannot be saved if we cannot manage to preserve our right to earn a decent living under conditions of equality and if we cannot exercise our right to make political decisions in the electoral arena. Therefore, what is necessary is a program of jobs with peace and affirmative action, democratic nationalization of basic industry and of the military industrial complex and the halting of racist assaults on Black people's political rights. This is the only framework within which practical programs addressing immediate problems of Black families will have any hope for success.

Observers of the current crisis within the Black family might find it instructive to examine the present situation in some of the socialist countries where there is also a substantial number of single-parent families.

In those countries there is no suggestion whatsoever of the soaring poverty associated with the growth of such families in the United States. There, however, the economy is crisis free, and, furthermore, if there are any social privileges to speak of, they are claimed by the youngest generations.

If, as Black people in the United States, we want to guarantee that the dream for a better life lives on through our children, and, indeed, that our children live on to see a better life, we must start learning to set our sights on a socialist future.

WHAT IS POLITICAL BIAS?

This activity may be used as an individualized study guide for students in libraries and resource centers or as a discussion catalyst in small group and classroom discussions.

Many readers are unaware that written material usually expresses an opinion or bias. The skill to read with insight and understanding requires the ability to detect different kinds of bias. Political bias, race bias, sex bias, ethnocentric bias and religious bias are five basic kinds of opinions expressed in editorials and literature that attempt to persuade. This activity will focus on political bias defined below.

5 KINDS OF EDITORIAL OPINION OR BIAS

*sex bias— *the expression of dislike for and/or feeling of superiority over a person because of gender or sexual preference*

*race bias— the expression of dislike for and/or feeling of superiority over a racial group

*ethnocentric bias—the expression of a belief that one's own group, race, religion, culture or nation is superior. Ethnocentric persons judge others by their own standards and values

*political bias—the expression of opinions and attitudes about government-related issues on the local, state, national or international level

*religious bias—the expression of a religious belief or attitude

Guidelines

Read through the following statements and decide which ones represent political opinion or bias. Evaluate each statement by using the method indicated below.

Mark (P) for statements that reflect any political opinion or bias.

Mark (F) for any factual statements.

Mark (O) for statements of opinion that reflect other kinds of
   opinion or bias.

Mark (N) for any statements that you are not sure about.

___ 1. Birth control is a legitimate health measure.
___ 2. The practice of birth control may be injurious physically,
   mentally, or morally.
___ 3. The practice of birth control is equivalent to murder.
___ 4. Birth control has both advantages and disadvantages.
___ 5. Only a fool can oppose birth control.
___ 6. Decency forbids the use of birth control.
___ 7. Birth control should be absolutely prohibited.
___ 8. Birth control is the only solution to many of our social
   problems.
___ 9. Birth control has nothing to do with morality.
___ 10. Birth control information should be available to everybody.
___ 11. Birth control is morally wrong in spite of its possible
   benefits.
___ 12. Uncontrolled reproduction leads to overpopulation, social
   unrest, and war.
___ 13. Uncontrolled reproduction is one fundamental cause of
   crime.
___ 14. The only salvation of the race is birth control.
___ 15. Birth control information should be included in every
   person's education.
___ 16. Birth control information should not be generally available.
___ 17. The practice of birth control is immoral.
___ 18. There is no justification for birth control under any
   conditions.
___ 19. There should be no restriction whatever on the distribution
   of birth control information.
___ 20. We should not only allow but enforce limitation in the size
   of families.
___ 21. Birth control is not a moral issue.

Other Activities

1. Locate three examples of political opinion or bias in the
   readings from chapter three.
2. Make up one statement that would be an example of each of
   the following: *sex bias, race bias, ethnocentric bias,* and
   religious bias.

CHAPTER 4

TEENAGE PREGNANCY: IDEAS IN CONFLICT

21   SOCIETY PROMOTES TEENAGE PREGNANCY
     Therman E. Evans

22   THE INDIVIDUAL IS RESPONSIBLE
     Joseph W. Tkach

23   CHASTITY AND SELF-DISCIPLINE IS THE
     ANSWER
     Mercedes Arzu Wilson

24   NEW SOCIAL POLICIES ARE NEEDED
     National Research Council

21 TEENAGE PREGNANCY: IDEAS IN CONFLICT

SOCIETY PROMOTES TEENAGE PREGNANCY

Therman E. Evans

Dr. Therman E. Evans made the following statement in his capacity as chairperson of The Mayor's Citywide Coordinating Council on the Prevention of Teenage Pregnancy in Philadelphia, Pennsylvania.

Points to Consider

1. Why is teenage pregnancy one of the most serious domestic issues facing the nation today?
2. How many children are born to teenagers outside of marriage each year?
3. To what extent is society responsible for this problem?
4. Why is there a lack of information on contraception?
5. How are radio and television networks involved in the issue of teen pregnancy?

The hypocrisy which revolves around sex in this society must be stopped. Our youngsters need their questions answered in an appropriate fashion, whenever they begin asking.

Teenage pregnancy is one of the most serious domestic issues facing this country today. This problem has serious implications and ramifications for the teenager herself, the developing baby, and the society at large. The implications and ramifications are medical, moral, educational, and socioeconomic. They include, but are not limited to, the following:

● Teenagers are more likely (17 percent of all births to teenagers) to have a low birth weight baby.

● Low birth weight babies tend to die within the first year of life, and if they survive, they may have physical and emotional problems that require years of intervention.

● Approximately 60 percent of children born to teenagers outside of marriage, who live and are not adopted, receive welfare.

● Many teenagers are themselves still growing and developing physically and psychoemotionally. Therefore, they are less likely and less able to properly care for a pregnancy and indeed an infant.

● Teenage mothers are half as likely to graduate from high school as women who wait until age 20 to have their first child.

● A study conducted at Attica State Prison in New York found that 90 percent of inmates were born to teenage mothers.

● Children born to teenage mothers tend to have low achievement scores and are more likely to repeat school grades than other children.

● Among 18-year-old mothers, nearly 60 percent have not completed high school.

● Of today's teenagers it is estimated that 40 percent of those 14 years and younger will become pregnant; 20 percent of those 14 years and younger will give birth; and 16 percent of those 14 years and younger will have an abortion.

● Divorce and separation are three times more likely to occur among teenagers than for couples who postpone to their twenties having a child.

146

Pregnancy and Poverty

A recent study released by the Children's Defense Fund shows that the incidence of teen pregnancy has a direct relationship to poverty and lack of education. It does not, as the rightists would have us believe, have a direct relationship to race or ethnic background.

The study points out that youths living in poverty feel that they have no opportunity, and therefore "sense that they have nothing to lose by becoming parents."

This bears out what many teenage parents themselves have said: having a baby gives them something to look forward to, something to give meaning to their life. Put more pointedly, teens with babies are victims not victimizers.

People's Daily World, October 1, 1986

The above occur in the context of significant involvement by teenagers in sex. For example, in 1981 over 1.1 million teenagers became pregnant. Seventy-five percent of these pregnancies were unintended, and 434,000 of them ended in abortion. Sexual activity among unmarried teenage girls aged 15 to 19 increased by 66 percent during the 1970s. Of the 29 million teenagers, 12 million (7 million teenage boys and 5 million teenage girls), or over 41 percent, have had sexual intercourse before age 19. Only about 8.5 percent of these teenagers are married. These statistics are accompanied by the results of many studies that point out that teenagers know dangerously little about conception and contraception. They tend to delay seeking information on family planning and/or pregnancy until long after they have initiated their involvement in sexual intercourse. Many of them labor under misguided notions that they will not become pregnant because of the "time of the month," "what they eat," "how they feel," "how they did it," and other even more foolish notions. This lack of information, I believe, is related to the problem of teenage pregnancy.

Lack of Information

At the crux of this lack of information, and the problem of teenage pregnancy, are the media, particularly the broadcast media. What is the connection? According to the census bureau the average American family has a television set turned on almost seven hours every day. Teenagers watch nearly 30 hours of television each week. They also listen to the radio for over 20 hours each week. By the time they graduate from high school teenagers have spent more time watching television than being in school. The broadcast media rank either just ahead or just behind peers and parents as the greatest forces influencing the values and behaviors of teenagers. Television programming is replete with sexual comment, innuendo, and behavior. One study pointed out that during one year of average viewing, Americans are exposed to approximately 9,230 scenes of suggested sexual intercourse, sexual comment or innuendo. Another study of sex on soap operas pointed out that television portrays six times more extramarital sex than sex between spouses. It went on to indicate that 94 percent of the sexual encounters on soap operas are between people not married to each other. On any given day television viewers are exposed to between 70 and 90 commercials. These commercials use sex (inneundo and direct suggestion) to sell cars, travel, soft drinks, wine, toothpaste, clothes, and almost anything else you can imagine. Additionally, it should be mentioned that the more than 20 hours of listening to the radio are filled to a large degree with sexually explicit lyrics of current pop chart songs. All of this open and explicit promotion/utilization of sex, in my view, represents the hypocrisy that is helping to produce a large part of the problem of teenage pregnancy. Why do I say this?

The very same television networks and radio networks that use sex to attract viewers, listeners, and to promote products, refuse to air announcements or advertisements for methods of birth control. This is the height of hypocrisy. It's okay for the teens to see it, see how good it looks, see how good it feels, hear how good it feels, learn how to do it, learn when to do it, learn under what circumstances to do it, but, they should not know anything about how to prevent the most important consequence of involvement in sexual intercourse, pregnancy.

Access to Birth Control

The easy access to birth control information and services is mostly responsible for the significantly lower teenage pregnancy rate in other industrialized nations of the world. In a study recently completed by the Allan Guttmacher Institute a detailed analysis of the behaviors and attitudes of six countries (United States, Canada, England, France, The Netherlands, and Sweden) suggests, ". . . the availability of contraception and sex education (in its broadest sense) has been effective in reducing teenage pregnancy rates in other developed countries . . .", and ". . . government was generally not directly focused on the morality of early sexual activity but, rather, was directed at a search for solutions to prevent increased pregnancy and childbearing . . . teenage childbearing is viewed . . . to be undesirable and . . . teenagers require help in avoiding pregnancies and births." The study goes on to give a sad commentary on the plight of the American teenager today. It says, "they have inherited the worst of all possible worlds regarding their exposure to messages about sex. The media tell them that sex is romantic, exciting, titillating . . . yet at the same time they get the message that good girls should say no. Almost nothing they see or hear about sex informs them about contraception or the importance of avoiding pregnancy." A specific example of the difference in teenage pregnancy rates between the mentioned industrialized nations is: for every 1,000 teenagers between the ages of 15 and 19, the United States has a birth rate of 96. This is compared to England's rate of 45. In France it is 43, in Canada, 44; in Sweden, 35; and in The Netherlands it is only 14.

Pregnancy Rate

The rate of pregnancy among US white teenagers, 15–19 years of age, is 83 for every 1,000 girls in that age bracket. This figure by itself places the United States above all of the other countries against which it was compared. Further, the rate among white teenagers is on the rise. However, it should be noted that the most devastating impacts of this problem are still felt directly in the black community. For example, black children living in single parent households increased from 32 percent in 1971 to 49 percent in 1980 and to 54 percent in 1983. The black teen parent is more often economically disadvantaged and therefore less likely to be able to continue her education, acquire job skills and have the long-range opportunity to become self-sufficient. Marriage is not usually an attractive alternative because the teen father is often in no better position to provide financial assistance. And so, with no means of support, welfare assistance is the choice for survival. Unfortunately, this choice for survival in the short run, too often becomes a pattern of life in the long run.

Hypocrisy

Our society can do better than this. The hypocrisy which revolves around sex in this society must be stopped. Our youngsters need their questions answered in an appropriate fashion, whenever they begin asking. All systems of the society need to be involved in providing these answers: the family, the churches, the schools, and especially the media. Again, I say it is the height of hypocrisy for us to continue to allow the implicit and explicit sexual references on the broadcast media, while simultaneously, the same media do not advertise, promote, discuss, or in any way inform the public about the responsibility aspect of sex. This involves informing people, particularly youngsters, about the life cycle, the menstrual cycle, the pregnancy cycle, conception, contraception, and anything else that will help improve the youngster's ability to make more informed decisions and to assume responsibility for his or her behavior.

TEENAGE PREGNANCY: IDEAS IN CONFLICT

THE INDIVIDUAL IS RESPONSIBLE

Joseph W. Tkach

Joseph W. Tkach is the publisher of The Plain Truth *magazine, the official publication of the Worldwide Church of God.*

Points to Consider

1. What is the price teens are paying for the irresponsible use of sex?
2. What role has society played with illicit sex?
3. Why has the "just say no to sex" concept been ridiculed as simplistic?
4. What choice has God given humanity?
5. Why is lack of self-esteem a major cause of teenage pregnancy?

The "just say no to sex" concept has been ridiculed as simplistic by some who apparently reason that premarital sex is not in itself wrong.

Healthy attitudes toward sex have probably never been more difficult for young people to acquire than they are today.

Yet, never before has so much information about sex been so readily available to youth. But how much of that information is reliable? And how much of it is accompanied by the guidance necessary to use sex responsibly?

The Price

The price young people are paying for the irresponsible use of sex is appalling. Some one million teenage girls in the United States become pregnant every year. Perhaps one half have abortions. The other half million give birth to illegitimate children. Countless teenagers suffer from sexually transmitted diseases. How many of these young people will be able to have a happy, productive marriage, not to mention future?

Society seems to have accepted premarital sex as simply a part of life these days. Supposedly responsible adults often say, "Everybody's doing it. What does it hurt, really? We just need to teach kids how to avoid pregnancy and VD." Somehow, though, sexually active teenagers, who lack self-esteem, just don't seem to be good learners when it comes to avoiding diseases or pregnancy.

One of mankind's age-old shortcomings is that we don't look at the result of our actions. What is the result of premarital sex? How does it affect one's future? How does it affect a future marriage? How does it affect personal relationships? How does it affect one's children?

Society as a whole has compromised with illicit sex to the point that many no longer care. Young people today have to assume that irresponsible sex is OK simply because too many parents, schools, clergy and people in government don't have the conviction or determination to guide them responsibly. Where is the leadership and guidance that a young, immature, impressionable mind needs in advance on matters that it lacks experience to know for itself?

Why should youngsters have to find out the hard way—through debilitating STDs, the shock of pregnancy, marriage-wrecking sexual delusions, emotional scars and wasted lives—that premarital and extramarital sex and homosexual activity have serious consequences?

Just Say No

The "just say no to sex" concept has been ridiculed as simplistic by some who apparently reason that premarital sex is not in itself wrong. Anyone would admit the above consequences are bad, but the cause of those consequences, premarital sex for example, is often considered acceptable, even something to be expected. "Look, they're going to do it anyway, so let's at least teach them how to avoid pregnancy," the rhetoric goes. We should ask ourselves, WHY are they "going to do it anyway"?

Is it so inconceivable that educating youngsters about a better way, a way that has no debilitating drawbacks, might just help avoid the destructive results of sex outside of marriage? Yet those who call such education "moralizing" wish to push their brand of morality on an immature segment of society too inexperienced to defend itself!

A Choice

The living God has not forced his perfect law of love on humanity. He has given mankind a choice. "I have set before you life and death, blessing and cursing," he proclaims. "Therefore choose life, that both you and your descendants may live" (Deut. 30:19). God has made his instruction book for humans, the Bible, more widely available today than ever before in history. Yet how many people today actually believe what he says? How many are willing to recognize the Creator as having authority over their lives? How many really believe that he knows what is best for them?

When you hear a teacher, or professor, or clergyman, a judge, a law officer, or government official or anyone else say young people should be taught that premarital sex is wrong, and that saving sex for marriage is the best and safest use of sex, you are hearing truth—truth based on God's own authority—right out of God's instruction book for mankind.

Young people can be taught the truth. With patient, loving instruction they can be shown the better way. If you are a parent, you can have confidence that such instruction is right for your child because it is based on God's Word.

Do young people respond? They certainly do! Response to last year's Plain Truth article "Are You Sure Everybody's Doing It?" showed us that most teens and even young adults deeply appreciate frank, clear guidance that helps them stand up to the strong pressures that could lead to disaster.

Lack of Self-Esteem

Experts correctly point out that lack of self-esteem is a core cause of teenage pregnancy. A sense of rejection and inability to deal with self-doubt make it unlikely a girl will say no to sex with a boy who shows her some attention. Adolescence is a difficult time from any perspective. It is a time when people need support and loving direction from those who should love them most—who should really care about their future happiness.

Parents, love your children enough to tell them the truth. Help them deal with the pressures. Give them support and encouragement. They need it, and they need it from you!

TEENAGE PREGNANCY: IDEAS IN CONFLICT

CHASTITY AND SELF-DISCIPLINE IS THE ANSWER

Mercedes Arzu Wilson

Mercedes Arzu Wilson made the following comments as the executive director of Family of the Americas. This organization is the recipient of a grant from the Department of Health and Human Services entitled "Fertility Appreciation for Families." This is a prevention service, national demonstration project, which will develop, test, and disseminate a comprehensive educational program to assist parents to become better informed and more effective in providing sex education to their children; teach adolescents about their fertility, the importance of protecting their capability for procreation, and encourage them to accept responsibility for their sexual behavior.

Points to Consider

1. What is the nature of the grant titled the "Fertility Appreciation for Families"?
2. How has the wide availability of contraception influenced the rate of teen pregnancies?
3. How many people believe in chastity and self-discipline?
4. How has sexual freedom and permissiveness influenced relations between the sexes?
5. What are the freedoms that chastity provides?

Excerpted from testimony by Mercedes Wilson before the Senate Committee on Labor and Human Resources, April 24, 1984.

There are a vast number of people in this country who believe in chastity, self-discipline, and marital fidelity. If 50 percent of our young people are sexually active, what about the other 50 percent who choose chastity and virginity until marriage?

The main purpose of our project is to develop a program for parents to enable them to be the primary sex educators of their children from birth to adulthood. We will also develop a curriculum for adolescents, ages 10 to 14, based on their developmental needs.

A standardized program will be taught in centers throughout the country and will be evaluated to determine its effectiveness to meet the needs of each area . . .

Contraceptive Information

Evidence seems to indicate that wide availability and knowledge of contraception have, in many ways, been responsible for creating this problem and increasing the number of teen pregnancies.

As federal spending on family planning increases, so do teenage pregnancies. In New York State, in 1982, 66,000 teenagers experienced pregnancy. About half had abortions. More often than not, the others dropped out of high school. Two-thirds of those will be on welfare in five years. Their children will be disadvantaged, too. They're more likely to have a low birth weight and a lower I.Q. and repeat at least one grade in school. As one of those young mothers put it recently, "We need help, and we can make it if someone says 'we can give you a second chance.' " There'd be no need for that second chance if those teenagers had availed themselves of a first chance—to avoid pregnancy. The legislature has approved $5 million contingent on specifics about how to spend it. The Governor deserves congratulations for a fresh approach to an old, and often tragic, problem.

The *Journal of Reproductive Medicine,* December 12, 1983, reported that more than half the women exposed to contraceptive information do not make use of that information. "A study of 1,000 women presenting themselves for first trimester abortion at a Preterm Clinic in Boston, MA found that 55.7 percent of the

Sex and Marriage

The fact that sex is meant only for marriage is not some sectarian religious belief. All major religions and civilizations have held that concept. Even those who tout secular ethics without a religious base can see that promiscuity is bad for children. This is the reason we have laws setting an age of consent. But under the guise of solving problems, some social engineers are espousing the practice of moral amnesia.

Tottie Ellis, *USA Today,* September 15, 1982

patients had not used any type of contraception for three or more months prior to conception. The remaining 44.3 percent were using some form of birth control, and hence, pregnancy was a result of contraceptive failure. Nearly all the women in the study acknowledged that they had acquired some knowledge of contraception. However, why they were not making full use of this information is not known. This confirms that teenagers are *not* using contraceptives, and that, therefore, massive contraceptive programs are a failure.

In Sweden, where sex education and contraceptives are available to all children in grade school, and where day care support is universal, premarital sexual activities are the norm. Today, Sweden has a divorce rate 60 percent higher than that in the United States. Half of all pregnancies end in abortion, and of those children who are born, one-third are born out of wedlock. It is often the girls that pay the highest toll as they are usually left with a child that they must take care of for the rest of their lives.

There are nearly 5000 family planning centers throughout the United States which provide "family planning" methods and provide or refer for sterilization and abortion. According to the National Center of Health Statistics, the largest group using family planning clinics are women under the age of 20. Over 73 percent of the under 20 women never used or did not regularly use any method of birth control before visiting the clinic. After visiting the clinic, 79 percent of these women adopted oral contraceptives.

Even with this extraordinary commitment to family planning and sex education, more than half of all teenage girls are sexually active. Each year, one of every ten teenage girls becomes pregnant. Throughout America, nearly one out of every ten people suffer from a sexually transmitted disease. Because of the increase in sexual promiscuity, the demand for contraceptive devices and abortion has steadily increased and so has government funding for them. Over $2 billion a year is spent to treat sexually transmitted diseases.

Permissiveness

Even with these statistics in front of us, and even with the divorce rate we all know about, there are a vast number of people in this country who believe in chastity, self-discipline, and marital fidelity. If 50 percent of our young people are sexually active, what about the other 50 percent who choose chastity and virginity until marriage? What are we doing for them? We feel that the government, by funding our grant, has taken a positive step to support and serve another section of the population—a section that chooses to reserve itself sexually until marriage.

Professor Armand Nicholi, Jr. of Harvard reports that "many who have worked closely with adolescents over the past decade have realized that the new sexual freedom has by no means led to greater pleasure, freedom, and openness, more meaningful relationships between the sexes. Clinical experience has shown that the new permissiveness has often led to empty relationships, feelings of self-contempt and worthlessness, an epidemic of venereal disease, and a rapid increase in unwanted pregnancies. They have noted that students caught up in this new sexual freedom found it unsatisfying and meaningless." In a more recent study of normal college students (those not under the care of a psychiatrist), Nicholi found "that although their sexual behavior by and large appeared to be a desperate attempt to overcome a profound sense of loneliness, they described their sexual relationships as less than satisfactory and as providing little of the emotional closeness they desired. They described pervasive feelings of guilt and haunting concerns that they were using others and being used as "sexual objects."

Dr. Joseph Santamaria, Director, Department of Community Medicine, St. Vincent's Hospital, Melbourne, Australia comments that "the sexual union is the most intimate of all human interactions and it contributes to the deepening relationship of a married couple. Within this union, procreation is a joint sharing in the preservation of the human species, and so intimate is this relationship, in its inbuilt power to share in procreation, that it is recognized as being exclusive of all others. Fidelity is essential to the continuing commitment of the spouses' life-long union. By its very nature, the sexual act is both unitive and generative. By excluding the generative function of sexual union, it opens up sexual activity to purely recreational purposes. Once sexual activity becomes purely recreational, it loses its total purpose; it is no longer unitive and no longer generative. It has become a source of physical pleasure with no true meaning to the lives of the two persons involved.". . .

Chastity and Freedom

The Fertility Appreciation for Families project, working primarily through parents, proposes to present to parents and to 10 to 14 year old children, knowledge and understanding of a future that contains for them self-esteem through positive accomplishment rather than self-disgust because of premature sexual activities that lead to venereal disease, unwanted pregnancies, loss of family trust, a feeling of guilt, and personal unhappiness.

To encourage young adults to use contraceptives is a course of action destructive to them, their futures, their future families, and the entire country.

There are many young people today that want to choose chastity as their premarital state, and seek supportive counselling. Because "freedom" is such a catch word used by those who are in favor of premarital sex, I would like to point out the freedoms that chastity provides.

1. Freedom from unwanted pregnancy
2. Freedom from complications of the pill and IUD
3. Freedom from venereal disease
4. Freedom from early sterilization from either V.D. or unwanted pregnancy
5. Freedom from complications of abortion
6. Freedom from forms of genital cancer

7. Freedom from the stigma and sorrow that befalls a family with an unmarried pregnant daughter
8. Freedom to explore cerebrocentric rather than genitocentric sexuality

"Nature has dictated that young people are physically able to reproduce as soon as they become teenagers. They must be taught that intelligence and self-control are essential. Total success in avoiding unwanted pregnancy, abortion, venereal disease, complications of the pill and IUD depends not upon further advances in technology, but upon a strong national program stressing the advantages of discipline."

TEENAGE PREGNANCY: IDEAS IN CONFLICT

NEW SOCIAL POLICIES ARE NEEDED

National Research Council

The project that is the subject of this report, "Risking the Future" was approved by the Governing Board of the National Research Council, whose members are drawn from the councils of the National Academy of Sciences, the National Academy of Engineering, and the Institute of Medicine. The National Research Council was established by the National Academy of Sciences in 1916 to associate the broad community of science and technology with the Academy's purposes of furthering knowledge and of advising the federal government.

Points to Consider

1. Why is adolescent pregnancy a serious social problem?
2. What attitude should people have toward contraceptive methods?
3. Who should share the responsibility for addressing the problems of adolescent pregnancy?
4. What actions must be taken?
5. Why is poverty closely related to the problem of teen pregnancy?

Risking the Future: Adolescent Sexuality, Pregnancy, and Childbearing, © 1987 by the National Academy of Sciences.

Because there is so little evidence of the effectiveness of the other strategies for prevention, the panel believes that the major strategy for reducing early unintended pregnancy must be the encouragement of diligent contraceptive use by all sexually active teenagers.

Adolescent pregnancy is widely recognized in our society as a complex and serious problem. Regardless of one's political philosophy or moral perspective, the basic facts are disturbing: more than 1 million teenage girls in the United States become pregnant each year, just over 400,000 teenagers obtain abortions, and nearly 470,000 give birth. The majority of these births are to unmarried mothers, nearly half of whom have not yet reached their eighteenth birthday.

For teenage parents and their children, prospects for a healthy and independent life are significantly reduced. Young mothers, in the absence of adequate nutrition and appropriate prenatal care, are at a heightened risk of pregnancy complications and poor birth outcomes; they are also more likely to experience a subsequent pregnancy while still in their teens. The infants of teenage mothers also face greater health and developmental risks.

Despite declining birth rates since 1970, adolescent pregnancy, abortion, and childbearing have remained considerably higher in the United States than in the majority of other developed countries of the world, even though the age of initiation and rates of early sexual activity are comparable. The most striking contrast is among the youngest teenagers: U.S. girls under age 15 are at least five times more likely to give birth than young adolescents in any other developed country for which data are available.

Teenage families with children are disproportionately fatherless, and most are poor. Teenage marriages, when they occur, are characterized by a high degree of instability. In addition, teenage parents, both male and female, suffer the negative impact that untimely parenting has on their education and the related limitation of career opportunities. Teenage parents are more likely than those who delay childbearing to experience chronic unemployment and inadequate income. Because these young people often fare poorly in the workplace, they and their

Attack on Family Planning

If you made a mistake and studied logic as a child instead of politics, you probably assume that a foe of abortion is a fan of family planning. After all, you reason, the best way to deal with an unwanted pregnancy is to prevent it.

Under this cloud of logic, you probably even assume universal support for Title X. That federal program funds family planning, serves some five million women a year, prevents some 800,000 unwanted pregnancies and some 400,000 abortions every year.

The reality, however—the political reality—is that Title X is under strenuous attack by those who insist that a vote for the family planning program is a vote for abortion.

Ellen Goodman, *The Boston Globe*, 1985

children are highly likely to become dependent on public assistance and to remain dependent longer than those who delay childbearing until their twenties. Society's economic burden in sustaining these families is substantial . . .

Panel On Pregnancy

With support from a consortium of private foundations, the Panel on Adolescent Pregnancy and Childbearing undertook a comprehensive examination of issues associated with teenage sexual and fertility behavior and reviewed what is known about the costs and benefits of alternative policies and programs to address these issues.

On the basis of two years of review, analysis, and debate, the panel has reached six general conclusions:

1. Prevention of adolescent pregnancy should have the highest priority. In both human and monetary terms, it is less costly to prevent pregnancy than to cope with its consequences; and

it is less expensive to prevent a repeat pregnancy than to treat the compounded problems.

2. Sexually active teenagers, both boys and girls, need the ability to avoid pregnancy and the motivation to do so. Early, regular, and effective contraceptive use results in fewer pregnancies. Delaying the initiation of sexual activity will also reduce the incidence of pregnancy, but we currently know very little about how to effectively discourage unmarried teenagers from initiating intercourse. Most young people do become sexually active during their teenage years. Therefore, making contraceptive methods available and accessible to those who are sexually active and encouraging them to diligently use these methods is the surest strategy for pregnancy prevention.

3. Society must avoid treating adolescent sexuality as a problem peculiar to teenage girls. Our concept of the high-risk population must include boys. Their attitudes, motivations, and behavior are as central to the problems as those of their female partners, and they must also be central to the solutions.

4. There is no single approach or quick fix to solving all the problems of early unintended pregnancy and childbearing. We will continue to need a comprehensive array of policies and programs targeted to the special characteristics of communities and to the circumstances of teenagers from different social, cultural, and economic backgrounds and of different ages. Because adolescents are not a monolithic group, they do not all experience sexual activity, pregnancy, and childbearing in the same way. Our broad goal is the same for all young people: that they develop the necessary capabilities to make and carry out responsible decisions about their sexual and fertility behavior. The strategies for achieving these goals and the specific interventions to carry them out, however, should be sensitive to differences in values, attitudes, and experiences among individuals and groups.

5. If trade-offs are to be made in addressing the special needs of one group over another, priority should be given to those for whom the consequences of an early unintended pregnancy and birth are likely to be most severe: young adolescents and those from the most socially and economically disadvantaged backgrounds. In many ways those at highest risk are hardest to serve, yet they are also the groups that have been shown to benefit most.

6. Responsibility for addressing the problems of adolescent pregnancy and childbearing should be shared among individuals, families, voluntary organizations, communities, and governments. In the United States, we place a high priority on ensuring the rights of individuals to hold different values and the rights of families to raise their children according to their own beliefs. Therefore, public policies should affirm the role and responsibility of families to teach human values. Federal and state governments and community institutions should supplement rather than detract from that role.

These general conclusions underlie all of our specific conclusions and recommendations for policies, programs, and research.

Priorities

The panel has identified three overarching policy goals, presented in order of priority, that provide a framework for our specific conclusions and recommendations:
1. Reduce the rate and incidence of unintended pregnancy among adolescents, especially among school-age teenagers.
2. Provide alternatives to adolescent childbearing and parenting.
3. Promote positive social, economic, health, and developmental outcomes for adolescent parents and their children.

For most young people in the United States, realizing fulfilling adult work and family roles depends on completing an education and entering the labor force before becoming a parent. Accordingly, our highest priority should be to help teenagers, regardless of the timing of sexual initiation, to develop the ability and the motivation to avoid becoming parents before they are socially, emotionally, and economically prepared. Despite the amount of energy and resources devoted to prevention strategies, however, some teenagers will experience unintended and untimely pregnancies. For those who choose to keep and raise their children, supports and services to promote healthy development, educational attainment, and economic self-sufficiency should be available. Given the potentially adverse consequences of early parenthood for the life chances of young people, however, there should be alternatives to childbearing and childrearing. Abortion is a legal option for all women, including adolescents. We acknowledge that voluntary termination of pregnancy is controversial, and for many in our society it is morally reprehensible. Although the panel strongly prefers prevention of pregnancy to avoid parenthood, abortion is an alternative for teenagers for whom prevention fails. Adoption should also be available to those teenagers who choose to continue their pregnancies yet are unable or unwilling to assume the responsibilities of parenting.

Reduce the Rate and Incidence of Unintended Pregnancy Among Adolescents, Especially Among School-Age Teenagers
The panel is unequivocal in its conviction that the primary goal of policy makers, professionals, parents, and teenagers themselves should be a reduction in the rate and incidence of unintended pregnancies among adolescents, especially school-age teenagers. Several strategies can assist in achieving this goal: enhance the life options of disadvantaged teenagers, delay the initiation of sexual activity, and encourage contraceptive use for teenagers who are sexually active. Unfortunately, very little scientific evidence is available on the effectiveness of programs associated with the first two strategies, and so we can only endorse the development, implementation, and evaluation of such programs. For the third strategy, the scientific base is much greater, and programs can be based on the demonstrated effectiveness of contraceptive use.

Enhance Life Options Poverty and hopelessness, which exacerbate many social problems, play an especially important role in the problems associated with adolescent pregnancy. Sexual activity and pregnancy among teenagers are not confined by race and income, yet the correlation between poverty and adolescent fertility is well documented. For too many high-risk teenagers, there are too few disincentives to early childbearing. Inadequate basic skills, poor employment prospects, and the lack of successful role models for overcoming the overwhelmingly negative odds of intergenerational poverty have stifled the motivation of many to delay immediate gratification and avoid pregnancy. Young people need a reason to believe that parenthood is inappropriate at this point in their lives and that their opportunities for personal and occupational success will be enhanced by postponement. Several possible interventions are aimed at indirectly reducing adolescent fertility by nurturing the motivation to prevent untimely and unplanned parenthood, in-

166

cluding life planning courses, programs to improve school performance, employment programs, and programs to provide role models for high-risk youth. . . .

Delay Sexual Initiation A second strategy for reducing the rate of teenage pregnancy is to help teenagers, both male and female, develop ways to postpone sexual initiation until they are capable of making wise and responsible decisions concerning their personal lives and family formation. Several interventions are aimed at helping young people delay sexual initiation, including sex and family life education, assertiveness and decision-making training, programs to provide role models to young adolescents, and efforts to influence the media treatment of sexuality. . . .

Encourage Contraception Because there is so little evidence of the effectiveness of the other strategies for prevention, the panel believes that the major strategy for reducing early unintended pregnancy must be the encouragement of diligent contraceptive use by all sexually active teenagers. Male contraception, as well as male support for female contraception, is essential. In light of the demonstrated effectiveness of contraceptive use, especially use of the contraceptive pill and the condom, in achieving this goal—

The panel concludes that use of the contraceptive pill is the safest and most effective means of birth control for sexually active adolescents. Aggressive public education is needed to dispel myths about the health risks of pill use by girls in this age group, and contraceptive service programs should explore nonmedical models for distribution of the pill.

The panel concludes that, to make this strategy effective, there must be continued public support for contraceptive services to adolescents, such as has been supplied primarily through Title X of the Family Planning Services and Population Research Act, Medicaid, and other federal and state maternal and child health programs. Such programs should minimize the potential barriers of cost, convenience, and confidentiality.

The panel urges that sex education programs include information on methods of contraception, how to use them, and how to obtain them.

The panel urges continued support for a variety of contraceptive service models—including private physicians—to reach adolescents. Contraceptive services should be available to all teenagers at low or no cost. Clinic service providers, whether based in hospitals, public health departments, private clinics, or community service organizations, should make efforts to improve the effectiveness of their programs by (1) enhancing their outreach efforts to encourage earlier use of contraceptive methods; (2) exploring more effective counseling approaches to encourage compliance; and (3) enhancing their follow-up of clinic patients to track their contraceptive use.

The panel concludes that school systems, in cooperation with various health care and youth-serving agencies, should further develop and refine comprehensive school-based clinic models for implementation in schools with large, high-risk populations.

The panel recommends the development, implementation, and evaluation of condom distribution programs.

The panel concludes that efforts should be undertaken to develop and test the effects on contraceptive use and unintended pregnancy of paid promotional messages for contraceptives that are directed at sexually active adolescents.

RECOGNIZING AUTHOR'S POINT OF VIEW

This activity may be used as an individualized study guide for students in libraries and resource centers or as a discussion catalyst in small group and classroom discussions.

Many readers are unaware that written material usually expresses an opinion or bias. The skill to read with insight and understanding requires the ability to detect different kinds of bias. Political bias, race bias, sex bias, ethnocentric bias and religious bias are five basic kinds of opinions expressed in editorials and literature that attempt to persuade. They are briefly defined below.

5 Kinds of Editorial Opinion or Bias

*sex bias— the expression of dislike for and/or feeling of superiority over a person because of gender or sexual preference

*race bias— the expression of dislike for and/or feeling of superiority over a racial group

*ethnocentric bias—the expression of a belief that one's own group, race, religion, culture or nation is superior. Ethnocentric persons judge others by their own standards and values

*political bias—the expression of opinions and attitudes about government-related issues on the local, state, national or international level

*religious bias—the expression of a religious belief or attitude

Guidelines

1. Locate three examples of political opinion or bias in the readings from chapter four.
2. Locate five sentences that provide examples of any kind of editorial opinion or bias from the readings in chapter four.

3. Write down each of the above sentences and determine what kind of bias each sentence represents. Is it sex bias, race bias, ethnocentric bias, political bias or religious bias?
4. Make up one sentence statements that would be an example of each of the following: **sex bias, race bias, ethnocentric bias, political bias** and **religious bias.**
5. See if you can locate five sentences that are factual statements from the readings in chapter four.

Summarize author's point of view in one sentence for each of the following opinions:

Reading 21 _____

_____

Reading 22 _____

_____

Reading 23 _____

_____

Reading 24 _____

_____

CHAPTER 5

ADOLESCENT PREGNANCY IN DEVELOPED NATIONS

25 TEEN PREGNANCY IN WEALTHY NATIONS:
    THE POINT
    Jacqueline Darroch Forrest

26 TEEN PREGNANCY IN WEALTHY NATIONS:
    THE COUNTERPOINT
    Robert G. Marshall

27 TEEN PREGNANCY IN WEALTHY NATIONS:
    AN ALTERNATIVE PERSPECTIVE
    Joy Dryfoos

25 ADOLESCENT PREGNANCY IN DEVELOPED NATIONS

TEEN PREGNANCY IN WEALTHY NATIONS: THE POINT

Jacqueline Darroch Forrest

Jacqueline Darroch Forrest wrote the following article in her capacity as Director of Research for the Alan Guttmacher Institute.

Points to Consider

1. What pattern do pregnancy rates follow in the developed nations?
2. Why is there a large discrepancy between the U.S. and other developed countries' pregnancy rates?
3. How is the use of contraceptives described in the rich nations?
4. What widely held beliefs about the causes of teen pregnancy are clearly refuted by the Guttmacher study?

Excerpted from Congressional testimony by Jacqueline Darroch Forrest before the House Committee on Energy and Commerce, April 30, 1985.

Thus, the six countries represent a rather varied experience. At one extreme is the United States, which has the highest rates of teenage birth, abortion and pregnancy. At the other stands the Netherlands, with very low levels on all three measures and a pregnancy rate one-seventh that of U.S. teens.

The purpose of our study was to consider why teenage fertility and abortion rates are so much higher in the U.S. than in other developed countries; and to see if anything can be learned from the experience of similar countries which have lower adolescent pregnancy rates that might help reduce unintended teenage pregnancy and childbearing in the U.S. . . .

Pregnancy Rates

The U.S. rates are distinctly higher than those of the other five countries; the Dutch rates are clearly lower. The French teenage pregnancy rates appear to be low among teenagers 16 and younger, and after that age to be high. The reverse is true of Canada. In the U.S., the pregnancy rates among black teenagers are significantly higher than those among whites, but even the white teen pregnancy rate in this country is higher than the rates for teens in other countries.

Thus, the six countries represent a rather varied experience. At one extreme is the United States, which has the highest rates of teenage birth, abortion and pregnancy. At the other stands the Netherlands, with very low levels on all three measures and a pregnancy rate one-seventh that of U.S. teens. Canada, France, and England and Wales are quite similar to one another, with pregnancy rates about half of that in the U.S. Sweden is notable for its low adolescent birthrates, although its teenage abortion rates are generally higher than those reported for any country except the U.S. and its pregnancy rate is about one third that of the U.S. It is noteworthy, however, that the United States is the only one of these countries where the incidence of teenage pregnancy has been increasing in recent years.

The Discrepancy

The next question we asked ourselves was: why this discrepancy between the U.S. and the other countries? Lower birthrates in other countries could result from greater use of abortion to terminate unintended pregnancies. However, the U.S. abortion rate is *higher* than elsewhere—indeed, the U.S. abortion rate is as high or higher than the overall teenage pregnancy rate in any of these countries—so the explanation for the high birthrates must lie in the determinants of teenage *pregnancy,* not in recourse to abortion. We speculated that more young women in this country might perhaps be *choosing* to become pregnant. But we found that a higher proportion of teen pregnancies in this country were unintended than in the other countries. About three quarters of teen pregnancies here and in Canada are unintended, as compared to close to two-thirds in England and Wales and France and only about half in the Netherlands. If only those U.S. teens who intended to get pregnant did so, our pregnancy rate would be 22 per 1,000 women age 15–19, compared to 96 per 1,000 today.

The variation in adolescent pregnancy rates also cannot be explained away by differences in levels of sexual experience. The differences in sexual activity among teenagers in the six countries do not appear to be nearly so great as the differences in pregnancy rates. The median age at first intercourse is very similar for the United States, France, Great Britain and the Netherlands—something under age 18—and is about a year younger in Sweden, and may be about a year higher in Canada.

Contraceptives

Data on teenage contraceptive use *do* indicate that the U.S. has the lowest level of contraceptive practice—which, of course, could help account for its high pregnancy rates. In particular, use of the pill—one of the most effective methods—appears to be less widespread among U.S. teenagers, possibly because of ambivalent attitudes toward the pill here—in other countries the pill is generally viewed as *the* most appropriate method for adolescents—as well as less easy access of U.S. teens to the pill.

Contraceptive services appear to be most accessible to teenagers in England and Wales, the Netherlands and Sweden.

174

The U.S. and Other Nations

The Alan Guttmacher Institute study shows that none of the other countries are hoarding some secret ingredient that keeps levels of teenage childbearing and abortion low: Universally available, confidential and free or low-cost contraceptive services combined with realistic and timely information about sexuality and contraception through the schools or the media are the common threads running through all the countries studied. What appears to be lacking in the United States is the political will exercised in the other countries to take necessary action.

The WREE View of Women, September-October 1985

In England and Wales and the Netherlands, those seeking care may choose to go either to a general practitioner or to one of a reasonably dense network of clinics. In Sweden, there are two parallel clinic systems, one consisting of the primary health care centers that serve every community, and the other consisting of a less complete network providing contraceptive care and related services to the school-age population.

Canada, France and the United States also have clinic systems, but these appear to be less accessible than those found in the other countries. The Canadian clinic system is uneven, with fairly complete coverage for adolescents in Ontario and Quebec, and scattered services elsewhere. The U.S. clinic network is reasonably accessible in a strictly geographic sense. Moreover, all family planning clinics receiving federal funds are required to serve adolescents. A basic drawback of the U.S. clinic system, however, is that it was developed as a service for the poor, and is often avoided by teenagers who consider clinics places where only welfare clients go.

Condoms are widely available in England and Wales, the Netherlands and Sweden. They not only are available from family planning clinics and pharmacies, but also are sold in supermarkets and other shops and in vending machines. In France and in many parts of Canada and the United States, condoms are less freely available.

Confidentiality was found to be an important issue in every country and teenagers were found to be able to obtain contraception without parental consent in all five other countries. (In Britain, however, the government is in court defending a policy of confidentiality for teens under age 16—a policy diametrically opposed to that defended by the U.S. government with its now-defunct "Squeal Rule").

Contraception is also generally available free or at very low cost in the countries we studied. The potential expense of obtaining contraceptive services in the United States, however, varies considerably. Indigent teenagers from eligible families are able to get free care through Medicaid, and others do not have to pay anything because of individual clinic policy; otherwise, clinic fees are likely to be modest. On the other hand, consulting a private doctor usually entails appreciable expense, as does purchase of supplies at pharmacies.

Information about sex and birth control also seems to be more widespread in the other countries that we studied . . .

Optimistic Study

I believe our study is a very optimistic study because, while it documents how far the U.S. still has to go in reducing the levels of unintended teenage pregnancy, it shows that it *is* possible and suggests ways it might be approached. Some widely-held beliefs about the causes of teenage pregnancy which have taken up research, programmatic and policy attention are clearly refuted by the evidence from our study:

● Young teenagers are *not* too immature to use contraceptives effectively, as evidenced by results from the other countries we studied;

● The availability of generous welfare benefits and services does *not* appear to be responsible for the U.S. having higher teenage birthrates than other developed countries. In fact, in all five countries, benefits are more generous than those in the U.S.;

● Low teenage birthrates in the other countries are not achieved by greater recourse to abortion—on the contrary, all have much lower teenage abortion rates than the U.S., but they have smaller proportions of teenagers getting pregnant in the first place;

176

- Teenage pregnancy rates are *lower* in countries with *greater* availability of birth control and sex education;
- Teenage pregnancy in the U.S. is *not* primarily a black phenomenon, since white rates alone far outstrip those of the other five countries, which themselves have sizable minority populations with often disproportionately high fertility;
- High teenage pregnancy in the U.S. cannot be ascribed to teenage unemployment, since unemployment among the young is a very serious problem in all the countries studied.

Government Actions

In all five countries we studied in depth, government actions have demonstrated a determination to minimize the incidence of teenage pregnancy, abortion and childbearing, though each has developed its own unique approach to the problem. In the Netherlands, the country with the lowest rates of any of the five, sex education in the schools is perfunctory, but clear, complete information about contraception is widely promulgated in all the media, and mobile sex education teams operate under the auspices of the government-subsidized family planning association. In Sweden, which liberalized its abortion laws in 1975, a concerted effort was made to assure that teenage abortion rates did not rise as a result, through increased attention to sex education in all schools and linkages between schools and contraceptive clinic services for adolescents, more so than in the United States, the pill is accepted by the medical profession as the most appropriate method for teenagers and is widely prescribed, often without the requirement of a pelvic examination. In all case-study countries, sexually active teenagers are more likely than those in the United States to use contraception and to use the pill, the most effective method. In all but the Netherlands and Canada, there is a national policy encouraging—in the case of Sweden, requiring—sex education in the schools.

Concerted Effort

Through a number of routes, with varying emphasis on types of effort, the governments of these countries have made a concerted public effort to help sexually-active young people to avoid unintended pregnancy and childbearing. In the U.S., by contrast, there has been no well-defined expression of political will. Policy makers, particularly, appear divided over what the government's primary mission should be: the eradication or discouragement of sexual activity among young unmarried people, or the reduction of teenage pregnancy through promotion of contraceptive use. American teenagers seem to have inherited the worst of all possible worlds regarding their exposure to messages about sex: movies, music, radio and TV tell them sex is romantic, exciting, titillating; premarital sex and cohabitation are visible ways of life among the adults they see and hear about; their own parents or their parents' friends are likely to be divorced or separated but involved in sexual relationships. Yet, at the same time, young people get the message good girls should say no. Almost nothing that they see or hear about sex informs them about contraception or the importance of avoiding pregnancy. Such messages lead to an ambivalence about sex that stifles communication and exposes young people to increased risk of pregnancy, out-of-wedlock births and abortions.

There are no easy solutions to the problem of unintended teenage pregnancy and childbearing and our study, while suggesting some directions, does not point to a magic bullet. If I could offer one recommendation it would be that we need some consensus in the U.S. on what the legitimate role of government should be in addressing the problems of teenage pregnancy and childbearing. Are we trying to eradicate premarital sex among teenagers? To reduce the incidence of teenage childbearing? Or to reduce the levels of unintended pregnancy among teens? It is in part the ambivalence about the definition of the problem and the government's role in addressing it that makes the U.S. problem so difficult to deal with effectively. If we wanted to pattern U.S. policy on that of the developed nations we studied, the focus of *public* policies and programs would be to prevent unintended teenage pregnancy and childbearing. The U.S. is the only country to have an official government program to discourage teenagers from having sexual relations and it is not clear whether that program is having any success. In Europe, by contrast, the morality of early sexual activity is a matter left to families, churches and other private institutions.

26 ADOLESCENT PREGNANCY IN DEVELOPED NATIONS

TEEN PREGNANCY IN WEALTHY NATIONS: THE COUNTERPOINT

Robert G. Marshall

Robert G. Marshall was the Director of Research for an American Life Lobby Report critical of the Alan Guttmacher Institute study of "Teenage Pregnancy in Developed Countries."

Points to Consider

1. How is the Alan Guttmacher Institute defined?
2. What is the whole report an example of?
3. Which approach is largely untried to prevent out-of-wedlock births?
4. What contraceptive usage-related plans are described?
5. How is the Charles Murray book *Losing Ground* described?

Robert G. Marshall, "Exposed: Guttmacher Institute Sex Study Flawed," American Life Lobby, 1985.

The whole report is an example of social science in the service of partisan causes, offering the veneer of scientific respectability without its substance or thoroughness.

On March 13, 1985, the Alan Guttmacher Institute (AGI), which is the research arm of the Planned Parenthood Federation of America (PPFA), released a study conducted over 18 months suggesting reasons why the adolescent pregnancy rate in the U.S. is the highest among 37 developed nations.

The report was released only two weeks before scheduled hearings by a House of Representatives subcommittee on the reauthorization of Title X of the Public Health Service Act. This is no coincidence since Planned Parenthood is the largest single recipient of Title X funding in the United States.

While AGI researchers examined statistical data from 37 developed nations, their findings, conclusions and policy recommendations were derived from a comparison of teen fertility and sexual behavior characteristics in Sweden, France, the Netherlands, England and Wales, and Canada with those of American teens.

Summary of Critique

The whole report is an example of social science in the service of partisan causes, offering the veneer of scientific respectability without its substance or thoroughness. If this AGI report were to be subjected to the juror's oath "to tell the truth, the whole truth, and nothing but the truth," the conclusions, publicized findings and policy recommendations would be significantly altered.

"Corrected findings," in fact, would be such that a request for more federal money to continue Title X could not be honored by a Congress seeking to save tax money or protect the traditional family.

The conclusions of this AGI report are understandable in terms of Planned Parenthood's institutional self-interest, though not supportable in terms of the public interest. It is utterly predictable that AGI, as a special affiliate of Planned Parenthood, would recommend "relaxation of restrictions on distribution and advertising of nonprescription contraceptives, especially the condom"

Judeo-Christian Beliefs

Encouraging contraceptive use ignores and undermines the Judeo-Christian beliefs of the majority of Americans, who still respect the Ten Commandments —i.e., sex outside of marriage is a sin—and are trying to instruct their young to do the same . . .

When will we believe enough in our youth and their inner fiber and moral courage to treat them with the respect they deserve: not as unreasoning, wild animals, but as individual persons with dignity, free will and the ability to master animal instincts instead of being mastered by them?

Mary Ann Kuharski and Anne Collopy, *The Minneapolis Star and Tribune,* November 29, 1986

in order to promote the acceptance of Planned Parenthood's own brand of condom.

The AGI recommendation that all teens be considered eligible to receive birth control is beside the point since any teenager in the U.S.—no matter how rich his or her parents may be—is currently eligible to receive tax-subsidized birth control.

Remaining largely untried in the federal approach to the prevention of out-of-wedlock births is that taken by the American Cancer Society for lung disease, the American Public Health Association for teen smokers, Alcoholics Anonymous for problem drinkers, Weight Watchers for overweight persons, by Congress in threatening highway funds to states that fail to raise their minimum drinking age to 21 by October of 1986, and by physicians with their allergic patients, namely abstinence. This would cost Congress and the nation nothing but good example . . .

Contraceptive Usage-Related Flaws

A glaring omission by the AGI research team is the failure to quantify expenditures for teen birth control per 1,000 teenagers.

181

No government or private expenditures for teen birth control are cited as a basis of comparison in order to determine, as opposed to merely claiming, that "teenage pregnancy rates are lower in countries where there is a greater availability of contraceptive services and sex education" (p. 60). No service statistics or clinic utilization data are even offered to attempt to substantiate the AGI claim that the countries compared had greater contraceptive availability.

And, where figures are claimed to establish pill usage, the AGI report notes, "The emphasis on pill use emerged more clearly from the interviews (conducted by AGI—ed.) than from *incomplete* (emphasis added—ed.) statistics on contraceptive use summarized in Figure 6" (p. 58) (i.e., for Great Britain, France, Canada, Sweden and the Netherlands—ed.).

Some subjective estimates are offered regarding the percent of sexually active women using contraception. But even here no standards of comparison are offered the reader to independently verify the accuracy of the claimed figures.

Additionally, in Figure 6 different bases of comparison are relied upon to "measure" contraceptive utilization among the sexually active (defined as having had intercourse at least once). The unequal categories of comparison are "used at last coitus," "use regularly," "use currently," and "used in last four weeks." Even looking at the footnote cited as a source for this supposed information, the reader is still left to guess as to how the claimed percentages were obtained (p. 63).

Public Ignorance

Although the Alan Guttmacher Institute describes itself as a corporation for research, policy analysis and public education, the institute depends heavily upon public ignorance to achieve its goals. In this case the AGI researchers state: "In Canada and the United States many doctors insist upon parental consent before they will provide contraceptives to minors" (p. 58).

Failure to quantify the percent of physicians in the U.S. who require parental consent before dispensing contraceptives leaves the reader and public policy maker with the dictionary-definition impression of there being "a large indefinite number" of such physicians who are by their actions increasing non-marital teen pregnancies.

However, AGI's own figures quantifying the matter state, in a different study note, that 73 percent (52,049) of all general family practitioners and obstetrician-gynecologists in the U.S. provide minors with birth control without parental consent.

Furthermore, AGI researchers provide no data on the number, percent or rate per 100,000 women, of physicians in the countries compared who prescribe contraception without parental consent. The report does claim that such doctors prescribe the pill without even a pelvic exam. Perhaps this last point is a veiled suggestion to Congress and state legislatures that the pill should be so dispensed here, at least in publicly funded programs.

In any case, the total number of physicians per general population in the countries compared is as follows according to the 1979–80 U.N. Statistical Yearbook:

Sweden (1976) 1:561, United States (1977) 1:569, Netherlands (1977) 1:583, France (1976) 1:613, and England and Wales (1977) 1:632. The reader has to ask just what real level of contraceptive inundation is possible if this physician ratio is reflective of the medical infrastructure necessary to achieve a high proportion of teens on a medically dependent birth control regimen. Perhaps AGI did not want to elaborate on what they could not explain except by resorting to preconceived belief that government birth control subsidies will decrease social problems associated with unmarried teen births.

In another finesse, the AGI publicists state in their report, "However, most family planning clinics in Canada and the United States provide services to young women without any such restriction;" i.e., parental consent (p. 58).

Again, by relying upon the adjective "most" in describing birth control clinics, the minimal dictionary definition of a majority or 51 percent comes to mind. The actual number of birth control centers in the United States which provide birth control to minors without parental consent is 4,765 or 93 percent of such facilities.

Again, no effort was made (or if made at least not conveyed to the reader) to quantify such clinics overseas and to estimate the number of teens utilizing them in comparison to the United States. To do so might have undermined any credibility in the "reasoned conclusions" of the AGI-Planned Parenthood partisans.

Although AGI normally restricts its public policy inquiries to matters pertaining to human reproduction, at least one finding in

AGI's present report relates to an area outside of its self-defined field of competence. The AGI report states:

"It is often suggested that in the United States, the availability of public assistance for unmarried mothers creates a financial incentive for poor women, especially the young, to bear children outside of marriage. Yet, all the countries studied provide extensive benefits to poor mothers that usually include medical care, food supplements, housing and family allowances . . . In those countries, however, the existence of considerable financial support for out-of-wedlock childbearing does not explain the differences between their teenage birthrates and those of the United States" (p. 60).

Losing Ground

AGI's conclusion, aside from being irrelevant, is at variance with Charles Murray's well-researched 1984 book, *Losing Ground*. It is not that unmarried teens get pregnant to obtain welfare benefits, but rather that there is an economic incentive to remain unmarried if a young girl or woman is pregnant and chooses to give birth rather than abort the child.

Murray, contradicting the AGI assertion, explains it this way:

"It is not necessary to mention changes in the work ethic, or racial differences, or the complexities of postindustrial economies, in order to explain increasing unemployment among the young, increased dropout from the labor force, or higher rates of illegitimacy and welfare independency. All were results that could have been predicted (indeed, in some instances were predicted) from the changes that social policy made in the rewards and penalties, carrots and sticks, that govern human behavior. All were rational responses to changes in the rules of the game of surviving and getting ahead."

Murray provides an example to illustrate his point about the economic rewards available to a young unmarried, pregnant couple in 1960 and after 1970 in terms of government benefits and what happens to those benefits if the couple marries.

Before 1970 no economic penalty in terms of public assistance benefits is incurred by marriage. After 1970 there *are* economic disincentives:

"When economic incentives are buttressed by social norms, the effects on behavior are multiplied. But the main point is that

184

the social factors are not necessary to explain behavior. There is no 'breakdown of the work ethic' in this account of rational choices among alternatives. There is no shiftless irresponsibility . . .

"There is no need to invoke the spectres of cultural pathologies or inferior upbringing. The choices may be seen much more simply, much more naturally, as the behavior of people responding to the reality of the world around them and making the decisions—the legal, approved, and even encouraged decisions —that maximize their quality of life."

Conclusions

If the Guttmacher study on teen pregnancy in developed countries started as an effort in serious scholarship, it became, over time, a poorly researched propaganda piece all the rationalizations of which were directed at a single goal—the acquisition of federal dollars. The AGI effort is a study in deception, because of its omissions as well as its superficial and fallacious comparisons in search of public support for federal dollars to "solve" problems largely of Planned Parenthood's own creation.

The AGI tactic is to survey the social wreckage which the Planned Parenthood Title X program has facilitated and furthered, decry it as a disinterested observer, then suggest that more federal handouts be given to birth control entrepreneurs to "correct" the situation. This social science shell game was described by Kingsley Davis, a population control enthusiast, who wrote in 1967 that social scientists "are not likely to arrive at solutions which go contrary to their own sentiments or which offend or deprive the groups to which they are committed . . . The perpetual confusion of social reform and protest with social science needs to be combatted."

Reputable medical publications as a rule submit their publications to a committee of peers for criticism. The Alan Guttmacher Institute submits its partisan efforts to a public largely unaware of the shallow basis and self-interested conclusions and policy judgments of the AGI report. And even members of the media are generally not equipped to take the time to examine in detail the accuracy and cogency of the claims before press time or the evening news is scheduled to begin.

As a consequence, the fourth estate will generally repeat what Planned Parenthood wants repeated in order to establish as policy assumptions those public myths about curing the "problem" of untimely teen pregnancy.

This present critique of the AGI effort rests upon an examination of only two of the references cited and a short discussion of items which AGI researchers omitted, and has pointed to serious errors in method, improper comparisons, invalid inferences and unwarranted conclusions.

Other Flaws

A more detailed inquiry would no doubt reveal other flaws. That any policy maker would place any credence in and his own reputation behind such flawed research can only be a testimony to the degree to which some individuals attempt to distort reality to fit what they wish to believe or to achieve.

The late Bernard Berelson, himself a population control enthusiast, wrote in 1969 that such behavior is characteristic of the "behavioral science man . . . a creature who adapts reality to his own ends, who transforms reality into a congenial form, who makes his own reality . . . When it is seriously inconsistent with his needs and preferences, he is capable of denying it. In his quest for satisfaction, man is not just a seeker of truth, but of deceptions of himself as well as others."

27 ADOLESCENT PREGNANCY IN DEVELOPED NATIONS

TEEN PREGNANCY IN WEALTHY NATIONS: AN ALTERNATIVE PERSPECTIVE

Joy Dryfoos

Joy Dryfoos is an independent researcher on the development of new strategies for the prevention of teenage pregnancy at the Hastings-on-Hudson, New York research institute.

Points to Consider

1. What do statistics on birth and abortion rates tell us?
2. How does the U.S. compare with other nations?
3. What was the nature of the Alan Guttmacher Institute study?
4. What factors are involved in lower rates of teen pregnancy in other developed nations?
5. Does sex education belong in the schools?

Joy Dryfoos, "What the U.S. Can Learn About Prevention of Teenage Pregnancy From Other Developed Countries," *Siecus Report,* November, 1985, pp. 2–7.

Whether sex education is provided in school by school teachers or near school by clinic sex educators, the study strongly supports the connection between the school and the clinic.

The fact that one in 10 American teenagers becomes pregnant every year is no longer a newsworthy item. However, the fact that this rate has extended over a decade since it was first brought to the attention of the American public certainly makes teenage pregnancy a subject deserving of further study. The general picture in the United States is that the proportion of teenagers who are sexually active has plateaued, or even decreased a little; marital births to teens have dropped significantly so that an increasing proportion of births to teenagers takes place out of wedlock; and the number of and rate of abortions have stayed the same for several years.

The most recent statistics show birth and abortion rates by age and rate for the United States. About 6% (62 per 1,000) of U.S. girls aged 15 to 17 had either a birth or an abortion in 1981 as did 14% (144 per 1,000) of 18- and 19-year-olds. The younger teens had about the same number of births as abortions, while among older teens pregnancies were more likely to be continued to births. White and black rates for both outcomes differ significantly, so that black youngsters were more than twice as likely to experience pregnancy as white youngsters. It should be noted at the outset that although births and abortions to very young girls (under age 15) receive a lot of media attention, they are a relatively rare occurrence. In 1981–82, about 28,000 pregnancies were reported among girls 14 and under; less than 10,000 resulted in births (Dryfoos, 1985). These births, however, may have more negative consequences for the mother, child, and family than births to older teenagers.

Other Countries

These statistics are important and take on even greater significance when compared to those of other countries. Such a comparison was first published in 1983 by Westoff, Calot, and Foster. Charles Westoff, Director of the Office of Population Research at Princeton University, has spent many years exploring the determinants of differential fertility in the United States. Using a unique data set from the Institut National d'Etudes Demographiques in Paris, Westoff et al. analyzed teenage fertility rates at the beginning and end of the 1970s for 32 developed-country populations. The rate in 1979–80 was higher in the United States than in every country but Iceland, Greece, Hungary, and Roumania. Because of the differences among racial groups in the United States, the white rate was compared to other countries as well, and it too surpassed the rates in every country but East Germany, Iceland, Yugoslavia, Greece, Czechoslovakia, Hungary, Poland, and Roumania. Rates for western European countries were one-fifth to one-half the U.S. rate and for Japan the rate was one-twentieth. What social, economic, and/or population policy differences could account for the extremely high rate of teenage fertility in the United States as compared to countries thought to be similar in culture and trends?

Guttmacher Institute

This important question led to a much more ambitious project, carried out by the Alan Guttmacher Institute (AGI) with the collaboration of members of the staff of the Office of Population Research at Princeton University. With support from the Ford Foundation, a two-stage study was conducted: First, factors thought to be associated with adolescent fertility were analyzed for 37 developed countries (referred to as the macro-study) and second, in-depth examination of the issue was directed toward five countries believed to be comparable to the United States (Sweden, France, The Netherlands, England and Wales, and Canada). The findings from these studies have been summarized in a recent article in AGI's publication, *Family Planning Perspectives* (Jones et al., 1985) and widely publicized through press conferences in New York and London and a press release that resulted in both news articles and editorials in hundreds of the nation's leading newspapers. The study findings have been rapidly diffused and heavily debated, and are providing a framework for more stimulating discussions about the issues surrounding teenage sexuality than we have observed in recent years. The U.S. researchers and their European counterparts have participated in dozens of "media events" such as appearances on the Today Show and the Phil Donahue Show. The researchers were invited to present their findings to the Panel on Adolescent Pregnancy and Childbearing of the National Academy of Sciences. A book giving a detailed account of each country study and presenting the statistical tables in support of the macro-study was published by the Yale University Press (AGI, 1986) . . .

The study contains a great deal of information on social, economic, and political variables that may explain the fertility differences. The authors highlight a number of factors that relate to the provision of contraception which they regard as the key to success: a centralized government with a strong commitment to the welfare of all people, backed up with policies and funds that give adolescents access to health services; a society in which there is an acceptance of the fact of premarital sex; and a view that accessibility of contraception is the means for reducing the need for abortion. In addition, adolescents in low fertility countries know that the state will support them whether or not they are parents, and this rules out the inclination to gain support through parenthood. While educational opportunities are probably greater in the United States than anywhere else, and youth unemployment no larger a problem than in western Europe, unemployed young people in the other countries receive more support for training and other benefits than do the unemployed youth of America.

Finally, the study arrives at the difficult issue of poverty. Does the prevalence of poverty in the United States explain the high

190

fertility rate? The authors point out that "poverty as it exists in the United States is essentially unknown in Europe." The economic leveling off that has occurred during the past several decades in Europe has resulted in a strong ethos that everyone is entitled to a reasonable standard of living. Only in the United States is there evidence of the "existence of a large, economically deprived underclass," although in England there is increasing turmoil among chronically unemployed youth, many of whom are members of minority groups.

Implications

What does this provocative study really mean? Should those of us who are concerned about the issue of teenage pregnancy be plumping for a welfare state? Or should we just go about our business, admitting that this country is too hetereogeneous, too conservative, too full of religious fundamentalists, too large, and too decentralized to even begin to put it all together?

The weight of the evidence, with all its limitations, rests heavily on Sweden and the Netherlands, which by their own definitions do fall into the category of "welfare states." Young people grow up in an atmosphere of trust and acceptance by their families and their society and, in return, most of them achieve adulthood by acting responsibly. The reward for this behavior is the assurance of social supports throughout one's lifetime, even when employment opportunities are limited. England and France follow this pattern of national commitment, social benefits, and openness about sex to a lesser degree, with more loopholes for local options, less consensus about the degree to which society should support individuals, and greater heterogeneity in the population. But compared to our country, in all of these places the message is more consistent; children do not grow up with such a dissonance between public and private morality.

Where does this leave the United States and, in certain respects, Canada? Can we learn anything from those relatively small, highly-organized homogeneous societies? After all, the teenage population in Sweden is just 2% of the size of the teenage population in the United States, which numbers slightly less than 10 million females aged 15–19. No matter the scale, these comparisons provide an excellent framework for national introspection.

The United States

First of all, this study makes it clear that unintended childbearing is a problem somewhat unique to the United States in comparison to western European countries. There are still people in the United States who think the problem has been overstated, taking issue with AGI's previous publications that broke the news about the "epidemic of teenage pregnancy." The study helps Americans see that not only do we have a problem, but we can learn something from other countries regarding what to do about it.

The major findings challenge this country to respond to two levels of directives. A climate has to be created that not only accepts the fact of premarital sex, but gives young people the equipment to experience it responsibly. For our country, however, this directive is complicated by the social conditions in which many of our young people live today. The compounding effects of poverty and minority status are grinding under a whole generation of young people whose options are severely limited by segregation, school failure, and lack of employment opportunities. For many of them, parenthood is about the only alternative they perceive, so that when pregnancy occurs, even unintentionally, parenthood is accepted as the hand of fate. So in addition to changing the sexual climate, we have to do something to alleviate the social and economic problems of the children in the inner cities and the Appalachias of America.

Major Social Change

Does this mean that without major societal change the pregnancy rates are not likely to decrease? We will never become a "Sweden," nor is that necessarily the solution. We can, however, recognize that changing the climate to be more accepting of teenage sexuality and improving the access to greater economic opportunity are not unrelated issues. What are unrelated are the advocacy groups that seek the goals of sexual responsibility and open opportunity. In the United States there are thousands of groups working for the betterment of children's lives. In the sex education field alone there must be hundreds of people who do consulting, lecturing, curriculum development, teacher training, counseling, and research, and run group workshops. But few of these people are connected to the thousands who worry about school achievement, employment training, welfare, family counseling, civil rights, etc., and those people in turn are also not connected with each other. What the AGI study suggests is a broad "package" of requirements: a policy favoring sex education, openness about sex, consistent messages, access to contraception, and more equitable distribution of income. This means that schools, health agencies, media, and welfare agencies have to be marching in the same direction, all at the same time. Just following one of these tracks will not have the same impact as putting together the whole package.

The "package" that emerged in Sweden and the Netherlands, and to a lesser extent in England and France, could only emanate from centralized governments who laid out policies and, as in Sweden and the Netherlands, made sure they were implemented. Nothing could seem more distant in the United States in 1985 than a centralized government that would promulgate the policies we support and then provide the funds and the personnel to implement these policies. Perhaps some time in the future we will see a government and a public that recognize the necessity for a strong federal role. In the meantime, we can try to make changes at whatever political levels are available to us. Currently in the United States there are a number of state and local governments that are ready to move on the issue of teenage pregnancy and willing to make the connection between access to contraception and access to opportunities.

Sex Education

For people in the field of sex education, this implies a broader scope of activity—entering into local coalitions with clinic operators, school personnel, civil rights leaders, and youth employment providers (and parent groups, churches, youth organizations, etc.). This combination of concerned people can bring strength both to the design and implementation of services for youth at the local level and to the articulated demand that the federal level show a commitment to the future of American youth through funding, legislation, policies, and leadership.

For those who are impatient with the more global issues, this study has some specifics to offer to the field of sex education, verifying what has been said over and over again. Teacher training appears to be an almost universal need. Even in Sweden concern was expressed about the capacities of individual teachers to deal with the subject of human sexuality in a comfortable way. From the point of view of an "outsider," the study seems to suggest that in none of the countries do the people who run the universities which educate teachers consider sex education as a serious subject. Teacher training in sexuality seems to be left to short-term workshops, in-service training, and summer courses that concentrate either on the basic facts or on communication skills but rarely combine content and craft.

Sex Education and Clinics

The study feeds the controversy over whether sex education even belongs in the schools. If we were to follow the Netherlands model, we would be urging our family planning organizations to develop educational teams to perform this function in clinics and youth organizations, and in schools when invited. For many communities in the United States, that quite accurately describes the current role of Planned Parenthood and other family planning agencies. Whether sex education is provided in school by school teachers or near school by clinic sex educators, the study strongly supports *the connection between the school and the clinic.* This is a very important principle and appears to be implementable even in the United States. Involving the media would move the campaign along a lot faster.

When one reads this study, it is easy to get depressed and embarrassed about our current situation in the United States. As Evert Ketting, a Dutch sociologist, commented at a press conference: "How can the richest country in the world allow a situation to continue that would not be tolerated in other countries?" That is a perplexing question, and neither the study nor this reviewer can find a simple answer to it. One slightly more optimistic view is that we look worse in the aggregate than in the disaggregate. In many communities, there is a high degree of consciousness about the problems of today's youngsters and a great outpouring of resources to try to find solutions. As has been suggested above, given the present state of our politics, these solutions will have to be generated from the bottom up rather than from the top down, at least for a while.

EXAMINING COUNTERPOINTS

This activity may be used as an individualized study guide for students in libraries and resource centers or as a discussion catalyst in small group and classroom discussions.

The Point

"My tummy hurts," a 16-year-old girl at New York City's Martin Luther King Jr. High School told the school nurse a few weeks ago. It wasn't hard for nurse practitioner Fran Combe to identify the girl's problem—she was seven months pregnant . . .

Fran Combe runs one of the USA's school-based health clinics that is authorized to advise teen-agers about abortion and prescribe birth control. In this case, it was too late for contraceptives . . . .

It's a big change to convert the school nurse's office to a health clinic, complete with birth control counseling. People always fear big changes. But as long as parents are consulted, we shouldn't fear school health clinics.

It is foolish and dangerous when a teen-ager delays seeking advice for seven months after she becomes pregnant. It will be just as foolish and dangerous for us to delay the help these clinics can provide. ("Schools Have Role In Birth Control," *USA Today,* September 15, 1982.)

The Counterpoint

This radical concept of installing sex clinics inside public schools to dispense contraceptives to unmarried teenagers is fueled by the argument that teen-agers are promiscuous anyway, and the schools should teach them how to avoid having babies. The phrase the clinics use is "responsible sexuality"; that translates into "be promiscuous without guilt and without a baby."

In many instances, educators are victims of the sex lobby. Liberal do-gooders are using the schools to promote their particular brand of morality—which is the old-fashioned immorality. The promoters of birth control in the schools are offering quick

195

fixes and simplistic answers. (Tottie Ellis, "Keep Schools Out of Teen Birth Control," *USA Today,* September 15, 1982.)

Guidelines

1. Examine the counterpoints above.
2. Which argument do you agree with more and why?
3. Social issues are usually complex, but often problems become oversimplified in political debates and discussion. Usually a polarized version of social conflict does not adequately represent the diversity of views that surround social conflicts. Do the counterpoints above oversimplify the issue of school based health clinics?

Appendix

Overview

The following information is reprinted from a report by the Center For Population Options. Given changing patterns of adolescent sexual activity, most developed countries articulate a need to help young people make responsible decisions and prevent unwanted pregnancies. There is little controversy about these objectives; however, there are profound debates about how to achieve them. Policies and programmatic approaches vary considerably.

Scope of Adolescent Sexual Behavior

- Adolescent sexual behavior has changed profoundly in recent years; for example, in Great Britain alone, from 1964–1974, the number of teenagers reporting first sexual experience before age 16 increased from 2% to 12% among girls and from 6% to 26% among boys.[1]

- The median age of first sexual experience in most developed countries has been steadily decreasing; for example, in Finland, it has decreased by six months for men and three years for women in the last 30 years.[2]

- As the age of sexual initiation drops, teenagers are constituting a larger proportion of those seeking family planning services, including contraception and abortion. In the United States, 449,000 teenagers received abortions in 1979, nearly twice as many as in 1973; nearly 1.5 million teens attended family planning clinics in 1979, five times the number as in 1970.[3]

Sex Education in Schools: Role of the Government

- All developed countries permit or mandate some form of sex education in public schools, although instruction varies from basic anatomy to comprehensive family life education.

- In the last decade, many countries have acted to create or change government policy related to sex education, often to make it mandatory. Countries currently requiring sex education in schools include Czechoslovakia, Denmark, the Federal Republic of Germany, France, the German Democratic Republic, Hungary, Iceland, Norway, and Sweden. Others have legislation pending. (It is important to note that political and ideological shifts in government can result in rapid policy changes.) [4,5]

- In other countries, the content of courses and age at which sex education may be introduced are determined by individual schools, as in Great Britain, and Luxembourg.[4,15]

- Countries which have no official policy but appear to permit sex education include Ireland, Italy, Japan, the Netherlands, Spain, and Turkey.

Policy and Programs in Selected Countries

GREAT BRITAIN
Statistics:

- Since the early 1970's, although the number of births to teens has increased, the teen birth rate has dropped: in 1972, 10 in every 1,000 16-year-old girls gave birth as opposed to 1976, when the rate was 7.8 per 1,000.[1]

- In 1976, 1.54 million people attended family planning clinics in England and Wales. In England 200,000 young people under 20, including 8,000 under 16 visited such clinics that same year.[1]

Educational Programs:

- Individual schools determine the content of sex education courses, if any; consequently, the amount and type offered vary widely from school to school.

- In general, little instruction is offered in nursery school, while 70%–80% of primary and secondary schools offer some form of sex education. By age 12, most students have received hygiene and reproductive physiology information as part of biology, health or physical education classes.[4]

- Many private organizations offer education, counseling or clinic services. Contraceptives are available over the counter, through private clinics, or free from doctors as part of the National Health Plan.

- Radio and television offer health education programming, which is sometimes used in conjunction with in-school programs.

JAPAN
Statistics:

- Increased sexual activity has quadrupled pregnancies among school girls between 1968 and 1983; in 1982 there was a 10% jump in teen abortions.[6]

- The abortion rate is one of the highest in the world, with an estimated two out of every three women having an abortion sometime in their lives.[7]

Educational Programs:

- There is little or no sex education in schools. Until the early 1970's, "purity education" to promote chastity was standard, since traditional culture strongly discourages premarital sexual activity.[8]

- Mass media and magazines are the leading sources of contraceptive information for women. These often sensationalize the side effects of birth control and may contribute to the exceptionally low level of use of modern methods like the pill and the IUD.[8]

SWEDEN
Statistics:

- The teen pregnancy rate peaked in 1974 at 70 pregnancies per 1,000 women aged 15–19; in 1980 it had dropped to 43 per 1,000, a 38% decrease.[9]

- Eighty-five percent of all teenagers in Sweden use the services of teen family planning centers by the age of 20.[9]

Educational Programs:

- In 1956, Sweden became the first country in the world to establish a mandatory sex education policy; although actual program implementation varied considerably, some sex education had been taught in schools since the beginning of the century.[5,9]

- All children receive some sex education, although the content and quality vary considerably among teachers and schools.[8]

- Sexual issues are addressed in the context of personal, ethical, and social considerations. "Fundamental" values (like equality of the sexes) are taught to all students, while more controversial issues (like abortion and premarital sex) are taught in a "value-free" manner encouraging responsible personal decisions.[9]

- The National Swedish Association for Sexual Information sponsors clinics and provides books, pamphlets, and other materials.[9]

New Approaches to Sex Education:
Program Initiatives in Developed Countries

Media and Publicity Campaigns

- The Soviet Union, in the mid-1970s, began columns on sexuality in magazines such as the widely-circulated (11.6 million readers per month) *Health*.[10]

- Since November 1981, the French government has sponsored a campaign featuring family planning messages by a famous actress.[11]

- The Rutgers Stichting in the Netherlands sponsored a month-long campaign to increase their clinic attendance. It was built around the slogan, "How do little hedgehogs do it? Veeery carefully . . .", and achieved a three-fold increase in clinic attendance by young people from 1976 to 1977.[12]

- The city of Toronto in Canada devoted a week in 1982 to the "Choice Not Chance" campaign, which was highlighted by youth troupe performances of dramas related to teen sexuality.[13]

Outreach Programs

- In England, the "Grapevine" project sent young volunteers to pubs and other youth meeting places to encourage them to seek counseling or to visit local family planning clinics. A similar project was later initiated in the Federal Republic of Germany.[12]

- In the United States, a project, now at the Center for Population Options, produced public service messages featuring rock and sports stars for use by teen-oriented radio stations.

- In the United States, hotlines, such as Community Sex Information in New York City and Choice in Philadelphia, provide personal but anonymous help for young people.[14]

- The Polish TPR targets specific groups like work corps, juvenile offenders, and the military; it provides special courses at students' summer camps.[12]

Youth Centers and Clinical Services

- The Door in New York City offers a wide range of services including employment counseling, sports, and free birth control.[14]

- Brook Advisory Centres in the United Kingdom strive to provide an atmosphere for counseling and medical services that is "non-establishment" and particularly comfortable to teenagers.[1]

- The French MFPF clinic model schedules regular times for drop-in visits and emphasizes group counseling and discussion.[12]

- In the United States, schools are beginning to expand their health program into school-based clinics which offer an array of medical services including family planning. Such clinics exist in sites such as St. Paul, Minnesota, and Houston, Texas.

References

[1] Cossey, Dilys, *Safe Sex for Teenagers*, 1978.

[2] Kozakiewicz, Mikolaj, *Sex Education and Adolescence in Europe, IPPF Europe*, 1981.

[3] The Alan Guttmacher Institute, *Issues in Brief,* January 1982.

[4] International Planned Parenthood Federation, *A Survey on the Status of Sex Education in European Member Countries,* 1975.

[5] Paxman, John M., *Law, Policy and Adolescent Fertility,* 1984.

[6] International Planned Parenthood Federation, *Open File,* July 29, 1983.

[7] International Planned Parenthood Federation, *Open File,* April 15, 1983.

[8] Coleman, Samuel, *Family Planning in Japan,* 1983.

[9] Brown, Prudence, "The Swedish Approach to Sex Education and Adolescent Pregnancy: Some Impressions," *Family Planning Perspectives,* March/April 1983.

[10] "Russians Sampling Sex Education," *The Washington Post,* December 21, 1975, p. B12.

[11] "Bilan encourageant pour la campagne publique en faveur de la contraception," *Le Monde,* October 3, 1982.

[12] *Approaches to Selected Groups, IPPF Europe,* 1979.

[13] International Planned Parenthood Federation, *Open File,* March 19, 1982.

[14] Kirby, Douglas; Alter, Judith; and Scales, Peter, "An Analysis of U.S. Sex Education Programs," *An Analysis of U.S. Sex Education Programs and Evaluation Methods,* Vol. I, 1979.

[15] Lief Duprez, ed., *Sex Education and Social Development,* 1976.

BIBLIOGRAPHY

This bibliography is arranged in three topics in the following order: general, pregnancy prevention, postpregnancy services, plus an annotated bibliography.

GENERAL

Allen, James E. and Deborah Bender. "Managing Teenage Pregnancies: Success and Failure in Two U.S. Communities." *Health Care Management Review,* 5:2 (Spring 1980), 85–93.

Burt, M. R. and F. L. Sonenstein. *Exploring Possible Demonstration Projects Aimed at Affecting the Welfare Dependency of Families Created by a Birth to a Teenager.* Washington, D.C.: The Urban Institute, July 1984.

Burt, M. R. and F. L. Sonenstein. "Planning Programs for Pregnant Teenagers: First You Define the Problem." *Public Welfare,* 43:2 (1985), 28–36.

Congressional Research Service. *State Programs for Teenage Mothers: An Informal Eighteen-State Survey.* Washington, D.C.: January 21, 1985.

Dryfoos, Joy G. "School-Based Health Clinics: A New Approach to Preventing Adolescent Pregnancy?" *Family Planning Perspectives,* 17:2 (March–April 1985), 70–75.

Edwards, C. J. and J. Balkin (eds.). *1985 Federal Funding Guide.* Arlington, Va.: Government Information Services, 1985.

Eisen, M., G. L. Zellman, and A L. McAlister. "A Health Belief Model Approach to Adolescents' Fertility Control: Some Pilot Program Findings." *Health Education Quarterly,* 12:2 (Summer 1985), 185–210.

Harris, David et al. "Developing a Teenage Pregnancy Program the Community Will Accept." *Health Education,* 14:3 (May–June 1983), 17–20.

Mecklenburg, Marjory E. and Patricia G. Thompson. "The Adolescent Family Life Program as a Prevention Measure." *Public Health Reports,* 98:1 (1983), 21–29.

Moore, K. A. and M. R. Burt. *Private Crisis, Public Cost: Policy Perspectives on Teenage Childbearing.* Washington, D.C.: The Urban Institute, 1982.

Mott, Frank L. and W. Marsiglio. "Early Childbearing and Completion of High School." *Family Planning Perspectives, 17:5 (1985), 234–37.*

National Center for Health Statistics. Monthly Vital Statistics Report. Advance report of final natality statistics 1978–83. Hyattsville, Md.: U.S. Department of Health and Human Services, 1980–85. Vols. 29–34.

National Center for Health Statistics. *Vital Statistics of the United States—1981.* Vol. 1. *Natality.* Hyattsville, Md.: U.S. Department of Health and Human Services, 1985.

Salmon, R. J. and R. W. Salmon. "Policy, Planning and Program Development: Case Study—Adolescent Pregnancy." *Socio-Economic Planning Science,* 16:2 (1982), 63–68.

Tena St. Pierre and Richard St. Pierre. "Adolescent Pregnancy: Guidelines for a Comprehensive School-Based Program." *Health Education,* 11:3 (May–June 1980), 12–13.

U.S. Bureau of the Census. *Fertility of American Women: June 1984.* Current population reports, series P-20, no. 401. Washington, D.C.: U.S. Government Printing Office, 1985.

U.S. Bureau of the Census. *State and Metropolitan Area Data Book, 1982.* Washington, D.C.: U.S. Government Printing Office, 1982.

U.S. Bureau of the Census. *Estimates of Poverty Including the Value of Noncash Benefits: 1984.* Technical paper 55, Washington, D.C.: U.S. Government Printing Office, 1985.

U.S. General Services Administration. *Catalog of Federal Domestic Assistance 1985.* Washington, D.C.: U.S. Government Printing Office, 1985.

U.S. Office of Population Affairs. *The Adolescent Family Life Demonstration Projects: Program and Evaluation Summaries.* Washington, D.C.: January 1986.

Wallace, H. W., J. Weeks, and A. Medina. "Services for and Needs of Pregnant Teenagers in Large Cities of the United States, 1979–80." *Public Health Reports,* 97:6 (November–December 1982), 583–88.

Wallis, C., "Children Having Children." *Time Magazine,* December 9, 1985, pp. 78–82, 84, 87, and 89–90.

Weatherly, R. A. et al. *Patchwork Programs: Comprehensive Services for Pregnant and Parenting Adolescents.* Monograph 4. Seattle: Center for Social Welfare Research, University of Washington, September 1985.

Zellman, G. L. "Public School Programs for Adolescent Pregnancy and Parenthood: An Assessment." *Family Planning Perspectives,* 14:1 (January–February 1982), 15–21.

PREGNANCY PREVENTION

Block, Robert W. and Sharon A. Block. "Outreach Education: A Possible Preventer of Teenage Pregnancy." *Adolescence,* 15:59 (1980), 657–60.

Blythe, Betty J., L. D. Gilchrist, and S. P. Schinke. "Pregnancy Prevention Groups for Adolescents." *Social Work,* 26:6 (November 1981), 503–04.

Darabi, Katherine F. et al. "Evaluation of Sex Education Outreach." *Adolescence,* 17:65 (Spring 1982), 57–64.

Edwards, L. E. et al. "Adolescent Contraceptive Use: Experience in 1,762 Teenagers." *American Journal of Obstetrics and Gynecology,* 137:5 (July 1980), 583–87.

Edwards, L. E. et al. "Adolescent Pregnancy Prevention Services in High School Clinics." *Family Planning Perspectives,* 12:1 (1980), 6–14.

Forrest, J. D., A. I. Hermalin, and S. K. Henshaw. "The Impact of Family Planning Clinic Programs on Adolescent Pregnancy." *Family Planning Perspectives,* 13:3 (May–June 1981), 109–16.

Furstenberg, F. F., Jr., K. A. Moore, and J. L. Peterson. "Sex Education and Sexual Experience Among Adolescents." *American Journal of Public Health,* 75:11 (November 1985), 1331–32.

Hill, M. F. and E. L. Ricks. "Teenage Pregnancy Prevention: An Atlanta Program." *Urban Health,* 13:2 (March 1984), 26–29.

Jones, Judith Burns, P. B. Namerow, and S. Philliber. "Adolescents' Use of a Hospital-Based Contraceptive Program." *Family Planning Perspectives,* 14:4 (July–August 1982), 224–25 and 229–31.

Kapp, Lucy, B. A. Taylor, and L. E. Edwards. "Teaching Human Sexuality in Junior High School: An Interdisciplinary Approach." *Journal of School Health,* 50:2 (February 1980), 80–83.

Kirby, Douglas. "Sexuality Education: Towards a More Realistic View of Its Effects." *Journal of School Health,* December 1985.

Philliber, Susan Gustavus and Elane M. Gutterman. "Playing Games About Teenage Pregnancy." *Evaluation and Program Planning,* 3:4 (1980), 237–43.

Ralph, N. and E. Edgington. "An Evaluation of an Adolescent Family Planning Program." *Journal of Adolescent Health Care,* 4:3 (1983), 158.

Schinke, Steven P., Betty J. Blythe, and Lewayne D. Gilchrist. "Cognitive-Behavioral Prevention of Adolescent Pregnancy." *Journal of Counseling Psychology,* 28:5 (September 1981), 451–54.

Schinke, Steven P., Lewayne D. Gilchrist, and Betty J. Blythe. "Role of Communication in the Prevention of Teenage Pregnancy." *Health and Social Work,* 5:3 (August 1980), 54–59.

Zabin, Laurie S. et al. "Evaluation of a School and Clinic-Based Primary Pregnancy Prevention Program for Inner City Junior and Senior High School Males and Females." Paper presented at the annual meeting of the American Public Health Association, Washington, D.C., November 1985.

Zelnick, M. and Y. J. Kim. "Sex Education and Its Association with Teenage Sexual Activity, Pregnancy and Contraceptive Use." *Family Planning Perspectives,* 14:3 (May–June 1982), 117–19 and 123–26.

COMPREHENSIVE SERVICES

Aries, N. and L. V. Klerman. "Evaluating Service Delivery Models for Pregnant Adolescents." *Women and Health,* 6:1–2 (Spring–Summer 1981), 91–107.

Badger, E. "Teenage Mothers and Their Infants." *Clinics in Perinatology,* 12:2 (June 1985), 391–406.

Bell, Carrolle A., G. Casto, and D. S. Daniels. "Ameliorating the Impact of Teen-Age Pregnancy on Parent and Child." *Child Welfare,* 62:2 (March–April 1983), 167–73.

Burt, Martha R. et al. *Helping Pregnant Adolescents: Outcomes and Costs of Service Delivery.* Washington, D.C.: The Urban Institute, February 1984.

Delatte, J. G., Jr., K. Orgeron, and J. Preis. "Project SCAN: Counseling Teenage Parents in a School Setting." *Journal of School Health,* 55:1 (January 1985), 24–26.

Delaware. "Social Services Block Grant/Jobs Bill Demonstration Program: A Comprehensive Approach to Reduce Welfare Dependency, Evaluation Report." Delaware Department of Health and Social Services, Division of Planning, Research, and Evaluation, New Castle, Del., December 1984.

Johns Hopkins Center for Teenaged Parents and Their Infants. *The Johns Hopkins Center for Teenaged Parents and Their Infants: Final Report, 1977–1980.* Baltimore, Md.: 1981.

McAfee, Marion L. and Marjorie R. Geesey. "Meeting the Needs of the Teen-Age Pregnant Student: An In-School Program That Works." *Journal of School Health,* 54:9 (October 1984), 350–52.

Miller, C. J. "Helping the Pregnant Adolescent Remain in School: The Continuing Education Program." *ANA Publication,* March 1984, pp. 27–29.

Mitchell, M. F. "Reducing the Risks of Teenage Pregnancy." *Mobius,* 4:3 (July 1984), 20–25.

Nelson, Kathleen G. et al. "The Teen-Tot Clinic: An Alternative to Traditional Care for Infants of Teenaged Mothers." *Journal of Adolescent Health Care,* 3:1 (August 1982), 19–23.

Polit, D. F. and J. R. Kahn. "Project Redirection—Evaluation of a Comprehensive Program for Disadvantaged Teenage Mothers." *Family Planning Perspectives,* 17:4 (1985), 150–55.

Polit, Denise, Janet Kahn, and David Stevens.*Final Impacts from Project Redirection: A Program for Pregnant and Parenting Teens.* New York: Manpower Demonstration Research Corporation, April 1985.

Ryan, Suzanne T. "Education or Welfare." *Illinois Schools Journal,* 61:1–4 (1982), 28–34.

Southwest Regional Laboratory. "Final Report: Impact Evaluation of Too-Early Childbearing Programs Funded by the Charles Stuart Mott Foundation." Unpublished paper, Los Alamitos, Calif., May 1985.

Taylor, B. et al. "School-Based Prenatal Services: Can Similar Outcomes Be Attained in a Nonschool Setting?" *Journal of School Health,* 53:8 (October 1983), 480–86.

Annotated Bibliography

Anastasiow, Nicholas J. "Adolescent Pregnancy and Special Education." *Exceptional Children,* v. 49, Feb. 1983: 396–401.

"Describes programs aimed at reducing adolescent pregnancies and programs designed to teach knowledge of child growth and development, child care procedures, and handicapping conditions to all students so as to help them become effective parents."

Barret, Robert L., and Bryan E. Robinson. "Teenage Fathers: Neglected Too Long." *Social Work,* v. 27, Nov. 1982: 484–488.

"A comprehensive review of the literature on teenage fathers is presented in this article, along with recommendations on how services to unwed adolescent parents of both sexes can be improved."

Burden, Diane S., and Lorraine V. Klerman. "Teenage Parenthood: Factors that Lessen Economic Dependence." *Social Work,* v. 29, Jan.–Feb. 1984: 11–16.

"The literature reveals that teenage mothers have high rates of welfare dependence. Factors that lessen the long-term negative economic consequences of early motherhood include deferment of marriage, support from the family of origin, increased education and career motivation, decreased fertility, and comprehensive programs for teenage mothers."

Dryfoos, Joy G. "A New Strategy for Preventing Unintended Teenage Childbearing." *Family Planning Perspectives,* v. 16, July–Aug. 1984: 193–195.

Advocates the development of a program to increase "the adolescent's knowledge and understanding of the consequences of early childbearing, and her recognition of the relevance of these consequences to her own life" as a means of increasing a teenager's desire to not become pregnant.

Ford, Kathleen. "Second Pregnancies Among Teenage Mothers." *Family Planning Perspectives,* v. 15, Nov.–Dec. 1983: 268–269, 271–272.

"Presents national data on the contraceptive practice of teenage mothers, pregnancy rates in the year following their first birth and the planning status of those pregnancies. Data are shown by race, age at first birth, income level and marital status."

Frank, Daniel B. "When Children Have Children." *Chicago,* v. 32, Dec. 1983: 212, 264, 281–283.

"Every year thousands of teen-agers face the responsibility of being parents: sometimes they're ready; more often they're not."

Gilchrist, Lewayne D., and Steven Paul Schinke. "Teenage Pregnancy and Public Policy." *Social Service Review,* v. 57,, June 1983: 307–322.

"Outlines what social science reveals about the scope and consequences of teenage pregnancy. The authors review the history of policies and legislation that have addressed the problem and summarize the complexities of public involvement in teenagers' contraception, unplanned pregnancy, and parenthood."

Johnson, Kay, Sara Rosenbaum, and Janet Simons. The Data Book: The Nation, States and Cities. (Washington) Children's Defense Fund, 1985. 228 p.

As part of the Children's Defense Funds' Adolescent Pregnancy Prevention: Prenatal Care Campaign, report presents "national facts and State rankings on prenatal care, infant mortality and adolescent pregnancy . . . state, Medicaid, and AFDC fact sheets, and the Surgeon General's 1990 goal fact sheets; and . . . general and summary statistics and table containing vital statistics."

Jorgensen, Stephen R., and Sharon J. Alexander. "Research on Adolescent Pregnancy-risk: Implications for Sex Education Programs." *Theory Into Practice,* v. 22, spring 1983: 125–133.

Examines what can be done in the educational system to reduce the rate and number of adolescent pregnancies.

Koenig, Michael A., and Melvin Zelnik. "Repeat Pregnancies Among Metropolitan-Area Teenagers: 1971–1979." *Family Planning Perspectives,* v. 14, Nov.–Dec. 1982: 341–344.

Finds that "half of premaritally pregnant teenagers who marry while pregnant conceive again within 24 months of the outcome of their first pregnancy; this compares with fewer than one-third of premaritally pregnant teens who remain single."

McCormick, Marie C., Sam Shapiro, and Barbara Starfield. "High-risk Young Mothers: Infant Mortality and Morbidity in Four Areas in the Uncited States, 1973–1978." *American Journal of Public Health,* v. 74, Jan. 1984: 18–23.

"In summary, the children of young mothers . . . continue to be at increased risk for death and morbidity in the postneonatal period as a result of maternal inexperience and the socioeconomic disadvantage characteristic of young mothers. The results of this study underscore both the increased health problems of the infants of young mothers and the limitations of the resources to help them and their families to cope with these problems."

Mecklenburg, Marjory E., and Patricia G. Thompson. "The Adolescent Family Life Program as a Prevention Measure." *Public Health Reports,* v. 98, Jan.–Feb. 1983: 21–29.

"The Program has two major thrusts: . . . care services for which only pregnant and parenting adolescents are eligible and prevention services which are aimed at preventing adolescent sexual relations and which are available to any adolescent. [Also] the Program is funding projects that demonstrate and evaluate innovative services."

Miller, Shelby H. Children as Parents: Final report on a Study of Childbearing and Child Rearing Among 12- to 15-year-olds. New York, Child Welfare League of America, 1983. 117 p.

Describes the characteristics of this particular portion of the adolescent childbearing population; and ". . . determine[s] whether and in what ways younger adolescent mothers differ from their older peers, in order to make informed recommendations for policies influencing programs and practices aimed at the very youngest of all parents."

Moore, Kristin A. *Private Crisis, Public Cost: Policy Perspectives on Teenage Childbearing.* By Kristin A. Moore and Martha R. Burt. Washington, Urban Institute Press [1983] 166 p.

Partial contents.—Prevalence of teenage childbearing.—The consequences of early childbearing.—Premarital sexual activity among teenagers: Prevalence and determinants.—Intervention points for reducing early sexual activity and promoting effective contraceptive use.—Teenage mothers and the receipt of welfare.

—. "Teenage Childbearing and Welfare: Preventive and Ameliorative Strategies." By Kristin A. Moore and Richard F. Wertheimer. *Family Planning Perspectives,* v. 16, Nov.–Dec. 1984: 285–289.

Gives the results of "The computer-simulation research project which compared the effects of seven hypothetical strategies, or scenarios, on the incidence and cost of welfare dependency among young women. These scenarios project a range of possible outcomes resulting from interventions to either decrease adolescent childbearing or break the childbearing-poverty cycle."

Morgan, Carolyn Stout. "Interstate Variations in Teenage Fertility." *Population Research and Policy Review,* v. 2, Feb. 1983: 67–83.

"The extremely wide variation among states in adolescent childbearing is examined using indicators that request high or low modernity, i.e., percent urban, percent fundamentalism, percent black, and region percent urban, percent fundamentalism, percent black, and region (South—non-South); the intermediate variables of factors affecting exposure to intercourse (percent married females 15 to 19); and the deliberate fertility control factor of induced abortion (the state abortion-to-live birth ratio)."

Morrison, Jack R., and Sherri Jensen. Teenage Pregnancy: Special Counseling Considerations. *Clearing House,* v. 56, Oct. 1982: 74–77.

"Outline[s] the health, social, and economic consequences for teenage mothers and their children."

"Predictors of Repeat Pregnancies Among Low-income Adolescents. *Hospital and Community Psychiatry,* v. 35, July 1984: 719–723.

"Found that girls' attitudes toward contraception did not predict contraceptive use. . . . The authors suggest that parental support of contraception plays a more important role in preventing repeat pregnancies than does the adolescents' reported attitudes toward contraception."

Rosenbaum, Sara. Providing Effective Prenatal Care for Pregnant Teenagers. (Washington) Children's Defense Fund, 1985. 90, 44 p.

Partial contents.—The problem of teenage pregnancy and its consequences.—The effectiveness of prenatal care.—Barriers that prevent pregnant women from receiving prenatal care.—Building effective prenatal care programs.—Financing effective prenatal care programs. —Children's survival bill.

Thomson, Elizabeth. "Socialization for Sexual and Contraceptive Behavior: Moral Absolutes Versus Relative Consequences. *Youth & Society,* v. 14, Sept. 1982: 103–128.

"Considers the possible intended and unintended effects of adolescents' exposure to the two dominant socialization strategies for preventing adolescent premarital pregnancy. [Discusses] the moral-absolutes strategy, which focuses on preventing premarital sexual intercourse among adolescents; [and] the relative-consequences strategy, which emphasizes the prevention of pregnancy among unmarried sexually active adolescents."

Wallace, Helen W., John Weeks, and Antonio Medina. "Services for and Needs of Pregnant Teenagers in Large Cities of the United States, 1979–80. *Public Health Reports,* v. 97, Nov.–Dec. 1982: 583–588.

"Comparison of the results of the 1979–80 and the 1967 surveys revealed that few large cities (only five) had added a special program for teenage pregnant girls and their infants in the interim 3-year period, even though the number of teenage pregnant girls cared for in the special programs continued to be small compared with the total number

For a related article by these authors on the survey findings see JAMA [Journal of the American Medical Association] v. 248, Nov. 12, 1982: 2270–2273.

Westoff, Charles F., Gerard Calot, and Andrew D. Foster. "Teenage Fertility in Developed Nations: 1971–1980. *Family Planning Perspectives,* v. 15, May–June 1983: 105–109.

Reports on "trends and variations in teenage fertility during the 1970s" for developed nations. Finds that western and northern Europe have decreasing rates of teenage fertility while those of eastern and southern Europe are increasing. Blacks in the U.S. and Japanese have the highest and lowest rates of those studied.

Zelnik, Melvin, and Young J. Kim. "Sex Education and Its Association with Teenage Sexual Activity, Pregnancy and Contraceptive Use." *Family Planning Perspectives,* v. 14, May–June 1982: 117–119, 123–126.

"Young people who have had sex education are no more likely to have sexual intercourse than those who have never taken a course. However, sexually active young women who have had sex education are less likely to have been pregnant than their counterparts who have had no such instruction."